GET STRONG

THE ULTIMATE 16-WEEK TRANSFORMATION PROGRAM FOR GAINING MUSCLE AND STRENGTH— USING THE POWER OF PROGRESSIVE CALISTHENICS

AL KAVADLO & DANNY KAVADLO

GET STRONG

THE ULTIMATE 16-WEEK TRANSFORMATION PROGRAM FOR GAINING MUSCLE AND STRENGTH— USING THE POWER OF PROGRESSIVE CALISTHENICS

Published in the United States by: Dragon Door Publications, Inc.

5 East County Rd B, #3 • Little Canada, MN 55117

Tel: (651) 487-2180 • Fax: (651) 487-3954

Credit card orders: 1-800-899-5111 • Email: support@dragondoor.com • Website: www.dragondoor.com

ISBN 10: 1-942812-10-8   ISBN 13: 978-1-942812-10-4

This edition first published in May 2017

Printed in China

BOOK DESIGN: Derek Brigham • www.dbrigham.com • bigd@dbrigham.com

PHOTOGRAPHY: Scott Bock, Cheyenne Coleman, John Du Cane, Mary Carol Fitzgerald, Neil Gavin, Dirk Jansen, Al Kavadlo, Danny Kavadlo, Grace Kavadlo, "Big Ronnie" Parisella, Michael Polito, Nick Polito, Robert Rimoczi, Erica Stella & Annie Vo

COVER PHOTO: Michael Polito

EXTRA SPECIAL THANKS TO: Rosalie and Carl Kavadlo, John Du Cane, Grace Kavadlo, Derek Brigham, Paul "Coach" Wade, Nick Collias, Michael Polito, Jeff Duenez, Adam RealMan, Mike Anderson, Annie Vo & Wilson Cash Kavadlo

Kavadlo Brothers "Brooklyn Strong" Banner by Coney Island artist-in-residence Marie Roberts (www.ConeyIslandUSA.com)

The Kavadlo Brothers are contributors to Bodybuilding.com, where portions of this work have appeared.

DISCLAIMER: The authors and publisher of this material are not responsible in any manner whatsoever for any injury that may occur through following the instructions contained in this material. The activities, physical and otherwise, described herein for informational purposes only, may be too strenuous or dangerous for some people and the reader(s) should consult a physician before engaging in them. The content of this book is for informational and educational purposes only and should not be considered medical advice, diagnosis, or treatment. Readers should not disregard, or delay in obtaining, medical advice for any medical condition they may have, and should seek the assistance of their health care professionals for any such conditions because of information contained within this publication.

– Table of Contents –

III - BONUS SECTION

FOREWORD

BY MARK SISSON

T he Kavadlo Brothers first caught my attention in 2010 when I saw a video of them treating downtown New York City like one giant pull-up bar. They were making some very hard moves look easy and making the whole thing look like a lot of fun. As someone who's personally made it my mission to empower people to take responsibility of their own health and enjoyment of life, I was impressed with how the brothers used their modern environment in such a primal way and were clearly having a good time doing it. I shared the video on my blog, Mark's Daily Apple, a few days later in my weekly "Link Love" post.

Not long after that, I became aware that Al and Danny Kavadlo were also exceptional personal trainers, when I came across a two-part article that Al had written on the subject of being a fitness professional. I shared both parts of that article on my blog as well.

Over the next several years, the Kavadlo Brothers would appear on Mark's Daily Apple numerous times, not only through links that I would share to their ever-growing body of quality content, but also as guest contributors. When Al released his first Dragon Door book and DVD, *Raising The Bar*, I was proud to give him my endorsement, and Al became my go-to guy for bodyweight training.

When the brothers released their book **Street Workout** a few years later, I came to better know and appreciate Danny's strength and wisdom, and gave that book my endorsement as well. I've been on board with the Kavadlo Brothers ever since.

In my **Primal Blueprint Fitness** ebook, I promote a bodyweight training program, as I've personally built my physique using primarily bodyweight exercises. Still, some people are skeptical about the efficacy of a training program that doesn't use any external weights for resistance. Is it truly enough, or just "good enough?" Can you really get big and strong without slinging heavy weights around?

It depends on what you mean by "enough," of course, but the answer is generally "yes." Bodyweight training is a legitimate option for anyone interested in building an impressive physique, increasing their strength, improving their athletic performance, mobility, and flexibility, and establishing excellent mind-body-space awareness. Plus, the ability to bust out some ridiculous moves on the pull-up bars at the local park has to count for something.

If you want to get as strong as possible, however, just doing more reps won't cut it. You need intelligent progression. Progression isn't just adding reps. Eventually, you have to make the exercises harder to keep getting stronger by adding weight or decreasing the amount of leverage you have.

And that's part of the reason why some people opt for barbells over bodyweight training: It's easier and far less humbling to add weights to a bar than to remove leverage from a bodyweight movement. In many cases, to progress in bodyweight means learning an entirely new movement from scratch. It's harder to quantify than weight training and easier to get stuck. But that doesn't mean it's not effective. In fact, the degree of difficulty required to perform some of the more intermediate and advanced bodyweight exercises *implies* their effectiveness.

This is precisely why **Get Strong** is such a phenomenal program. In this book, the Kavadlo Brothers will guide you from the very beginning and help you build a proper foundation. From there, they'll gradually progress you through four phases of strength, giving you the proper progressions and programing details to take you beyond what you ever thought possible. The brothers have also outdone themselves with their incredible visuals this time, adding some primal scenery to their usual urban jungle aesthetic. This book is packed with well thought-out, clearly delivered programming and beautiful imagery.

If you doubt the effectiveness of a pure bodyweight strength training program, then I challenge you to follow this program for 16 weeks and get back to me.

Primally Yours,

Mark Sisson

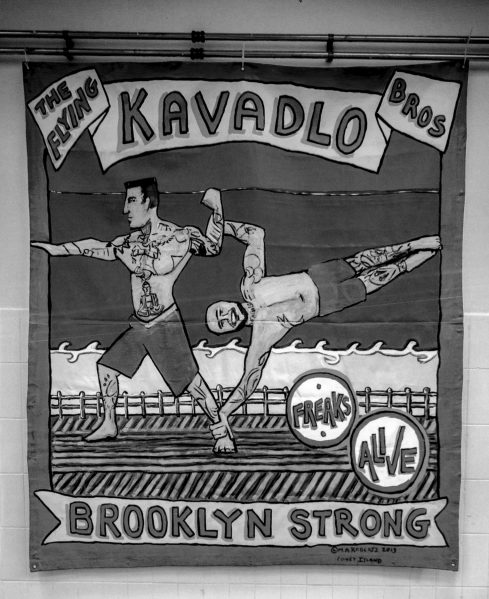

PREFACE

I t was 12 degrees Fahrenheit when we stepped off the plane in Beijing to teach Asia's first-ever Progressive Calisthenics Certification. A mix of energy, excitement and anticipation filled us.

We've had the honor of teaching the Progressive Calisthenics Certification (PCC) since its inception and it is the #1 bodyweight strength training certification in the world.

Though the PCC had already been going strong in North America, Europe and Australia, we were nervous yet also enthusiastic for our first foray to the Far East. It was our premier event of 2016, and we wanted to get the year off to a strong start.

After 16 hours on a plane, we arrived at Peking International Airport the night before the 3-day certification was set to commence. Sometimes our schedules allow us to spend some downtime in a new city before instructing a workshop, but this time that was not the case.

After making our way through customs, our hosts picked us up and drove us to our hotel, where we quickly checked in, dropped off our belongings and immediately made our way to dinner. We were taken to the most authentic Chinese restaurant we'd ever been, where we dined on Peking duck, spicy sea cucumber and squid. We drank ancient Chinese yellow wine brewed by monks, alongside Dragon Door CEO John Du Cane and several executives from Beijing Science and Technology Publishing, the company behind the Chinese translations of many bestselling Dragon Door titles. It was one of the most delicious and unique culinary experiences we've ever had.

The next morning, we made our way across the bustling cityscape. There was boundless energy and people everywhere. Finally, we arrived at the training facility, not knowing exactly what to expect. We were tired, disoriented and cold, yet once the energy of the 40+ calisthenics fanatics who showed up to train with us began pouring into the room, the jetlag, language barrier and pandemonium were no longer of consequence. As always, we delivered our signature blend of calisthenics coaching while the attendees set personal bests and forged new friendships.

It's amazing how the modern bodyweight strength training movement is still growing every day and spreading to reach more people all over the world. Though we are all different and unique, calisthenics continually reminds us that we have so much in common, despite our geographic separation and perceived cultural divisions.

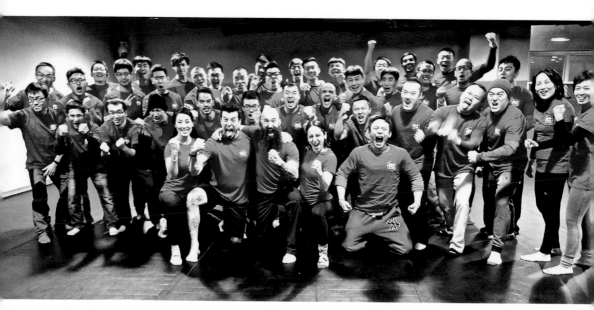

Later in 2016 we would travel to London, Munich, Amsterdam, Sydney and back to Beijing. We taught across the US multiple times as well. In each city and at every workshop, there is tremendous enthusiasm and energy, and we always have an unforgettable experience. Calisthenics has an incredible way of strengthening the body, but it also does wonders for the spirit. Bodyweight movement provides an opportunity for growth in many ways.

The world is starting to feel smaller, but the posse keeps getting bigger.

Across our travels, one of the most frequently asked questions we receive is how to put together a definitive program to build muscle and strength. Though many of our previous books have featured step-by-step progressions and numerous workout templates, the book in your hands is the very first to contain a detailed, actionable, 16-week training program, including specific exercise sequences, exact sets and reps, specified time frames, warm-ups and rest days.

You asked for it. You got it!

Get Strong is divided into three sections. The first, simply entitled *Get Strong*, includes the techniques, exercises and programs necessary to build a lifetime of strength. To anyone who's ever asked where the best place to get started is, or how far you can go, this is for you.

The second part, *Stay Strong*, consists of practical answers to real questions (Ask Al) and time-tested advice for fitness and life (Danny's Dos and Don'ts). Additionally, we've provided more exercises, workouts and even partner drills to supplement what you've already achieved in the first part.

Finally, the *Bonus Section* features ten of the best articles we've ever written, along with never before seen authors' insights. For example, if you are curious about breathing techniques, look no further than "Strength from Within." For the Kavadlo approach to nutrition (and making your gains more visible), you will want to check out "Six Tips For A Six Pack." The wisdom contained in these pages will support and enhance your journey, as well as provide unique perspective for future training endeavors.

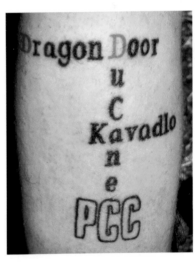

We've gone from being two kids in deep Brooklyn having push-up contests on the linoleum floor, to becoming renowned fitness experts across the globe. There are Kavadlo Brothers books available worldwide in over a dozen languages, as well as DVDs, T-shirts and apps for your smart phone. There are even a few "Kavadlo" tattoos floating around out there. We are grateful to every one of you for all of this.

From the bottom of our hearts, you mean as much to us as we do to you. Thank you for what you've given us. This is our attempt to give something back.

Hey hey hey! Keep the dream alive!

Al Kavadlo   D Kavadlo

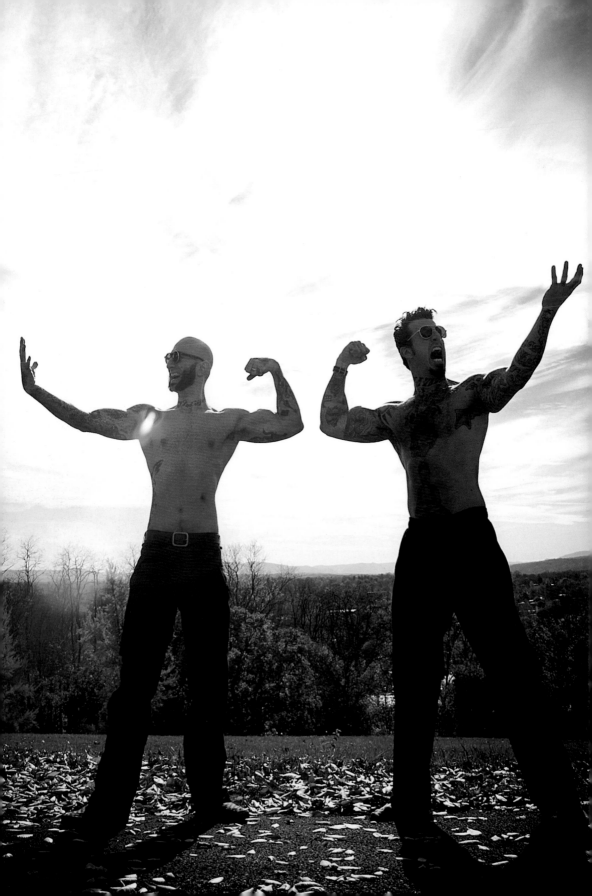

- I -

GET
STRONG

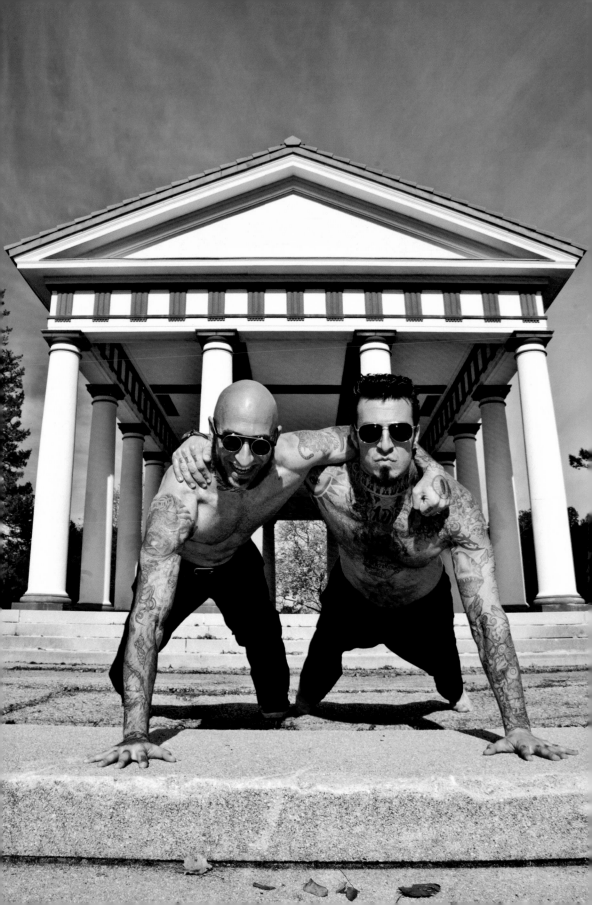

BUILDING YOUR NEW HOME

I f you were looking for a new home, but you didn't have a lot of spare time, you might hire a real estate broker to assist you. They would listen to what you wanted in a dwelling, and arrange to show you only the best options. Most of the legwork would be done for you, saving you time, effort and stress.

With this program, we have done the same thing for you, except with exercise. Just as a good real estate broker knows the best places in your neighborhood, we know exactly how to give you a challenging and effective workout without wasting time. We've done the legwork for you. Though not literally of course—you still need to do those squats yourself.

And just like that real estate agent would ideally save you both time and money in the big picture (time is money after all, right?), this book is a valuable investment in your health that can save you from wasting time with ineffective training methods.

However, unlike the broker, we are not merely seeking a new house. Not by a long shot. We are building the very vessel you *live in all the time*—your own body! That's right, this is more than just an address to which your mail gets sent or a place where you store your belongings. You don't just lay your head down at night and eat your meals here; you do every single activity of your life within the confines of your own skin. You use your body when you move throughout the world, travel to work, spend time with your family or do anything else.

We will help you build the strongest body possible. This will improve every facet of your life forever.

OCKHAM'S WORKOUT

"IT IS VAIN TO DO WITH MORE WHAT CAN BE DONE WITH FEWER."
-WILLIAM OF OCKHAM

There's a concept in science and philosophy known as "Ockham's Razor" which states that among competing theories, the simplest explanation is the most likely to be true.

We believe a similar thing about exercise: In fitness, the simplest workout program is the one that's most likely to deliver results. It's also much more likely that you'll actually do it.

There are many competing theories when it comes to training, and some are more complicated than others. Complicated, however, does not mean better. If the program you seek is the most stripped-down, efficient path available, then you are in the right place. What follows are the most direct methods for building strength and muscle.

All you'll need to do these workouts is a floor, a wall, a bench (or other elevated surface of approximately knee height) and an overhead bar (or something else you can hang from). This program does not require any external weights or machines. We won't be doing any flashy moves that require a ton of technique or precision either. Only the essentials for getting brutally strong and muscular.

You can go to the park, train at the gym or do these workouts in your home. As long as you get the reps done, we'll leave the location up to you.

PROGRESSIVE OVERLOAD

All types of strength training operate under the same principle of progressive overload. The only way to get stronger is to learn a movement pattern under a relatively low amount of resistance, then gradually increase the load and/or quantity of repetitions as the body adapts.

In weight training, this is typically done by using a relatively light weight in order to learn proper technique before progressing to heavier lifts. Due to the nature of bodyweight training, however, progress must be approached a bit differently. Since you cannot alter your body's mass as easily as adding or removing plates from a barbell, we instead utilize the principles of progressive calisthenics in order to adjust the resistance.

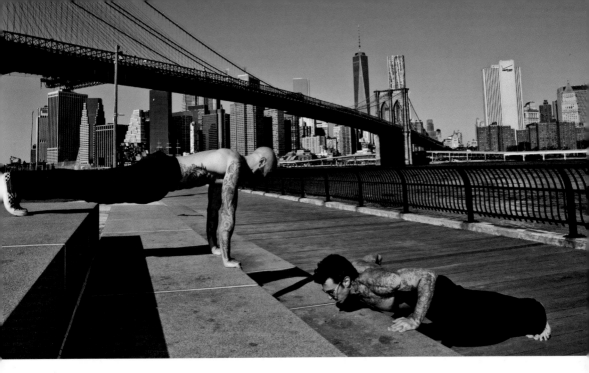

One way is to change the weight-to-limb ratio, which can be achieved by placing more (or less) of our weight in our hands or feet. To illustrate this, compare a push-up with your feet on an elevated surface to a push-up with all your limbs on the ground. Due to the change in leverage, there is much more weight in the chest, arms and shoulders in the former than in the latter, rendering it more difficult. Conversely, a push-up with the hands elevated (instead of the feet) will place less demand on the muscles of the upper body.

Another way to progress your training is to remove contact points entirely. A one-legged squat will always require more strength than a standard two-legged squat. By eliminating one point of contact, we've doubled the weight loaded onto the individual leg. Fortunately, there are many steps in between the two, such as the step-up or Bulgarian split squat.

Finally, we can alter the range of motion. One example of this is to progress from a hanging leg raise where your legs end up parallel to the ground, to a leg raise where your toes go all the way to the bar. The increased distance makes it harder.

THE *GET STRONG* PROGRAM

We've both been workout enthusiasts for most of our lives and we've been fitness pros for many years. We've trained thousands of clients in one-on-one, small group and large workshop formats. We've worked with the full spectrum of physical specimens, from 80-year old grandmothers with arthritis, to dancers, models and athletes—even Olympic medalists.

The exercise selection and programing decisions in this book reflect our own personal experience as workout practitioners, as well as our observations as trainers and coaches. These exercises are the most effective and efficient choices, and the progressions are the most universal and approachable.

This is the ultimate bang-for-your-buck bodyweight program. It is divided into four phases. Each phase is four weeks long and includes a week-by-week template of which exercises are to be performed and how many repetitions are required before moving ahead. We've also included a general warm-up, which you will perform at the start of every training session. If you stick to the program, you will gradually build your total repetitions of each exercise week after week as you experience increases in strength, muscle and body control.

During Phase 1 and Phase 2, you'll be doing full body strength training workouts three times a week, with at least one day of rest between each training session. These workouts should not require more than 50 minutes of your time, and in many cases will require less.

During Phase 3 and Phase 4, you'll be doing four workouts per week, following a split routine. This means you will emphasize different body parts on different days. There will be two workouts that emphasize the upper-body and two workouts that emphasize the lower-body during these phases. The purpose of the split routine is to allow for more total training volume per body part without increasing the total time of each individual training session. It also allows for additional recovery time, as you will be training each body part twice per week instead of three times. Again, these workouts should not require more than 50 minutes of your time, and may require less. Furthermore, by adding a fourth training day during the final two phases, you will now have more days that you are training than days in which you are not.

We encourage you to get additional exercise on your non-strength training days during all phases of the program. Activities such as walking, running, cycling and jumping rope are excellent choices. In other words, a "rest" day does not mean you do not get off the couch. But for the purposes of building muscle and unlocking your strength potential, this system is all you'll need.

Each phase progressively introduces more difficult variations on previous movements. New families of exercises are included in the later phases as well. At the end of each four-week phase, there is a test to assess if you are ready to move to the next phase and advance to more challenging exercises.

Here's a breakdown of what to expect:

PHASE 1—THE FOUNDATION consists of laying down the bedrock to prepare you for what's ahead. This phase is aimed at the beginner, and is not necessarily a requirement for everybody. If you're new to calisthenics or are returning to fitness after a hiatus, then this is where you start.

PHASE 2—BRICK AND MORTAR builds upon that foundation by bringing in many of the classic exercises that put calisthenics on the map. These are the basic components you need in order to construct your framework. Start here if you already have a solid foundation.

PHASE 3—CONCRETE AND IRON takes you into the realm of beastly strength. With the furnishings detailed in this section, your structure will be reinforced to weather the toughest of elements. Complete this phase and you will have more strength than most will ever achieve in this lifetime.

PHASE 4—FORGED FROM STEEL is comprised of tools and tactics for the advanced architect of the human body. These workouts are not for the faint of heart. Complete this phase and you will be amongst the elite in pound-for-pound strength.

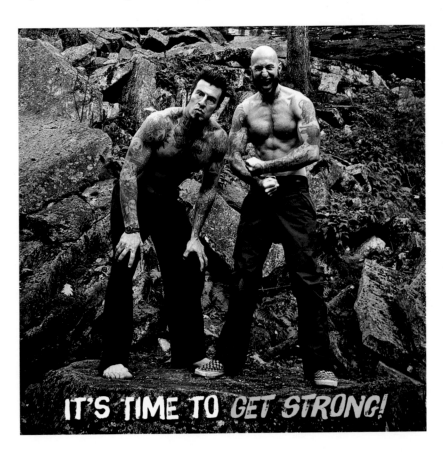

IT'S TIME TO *GET STRONG!*

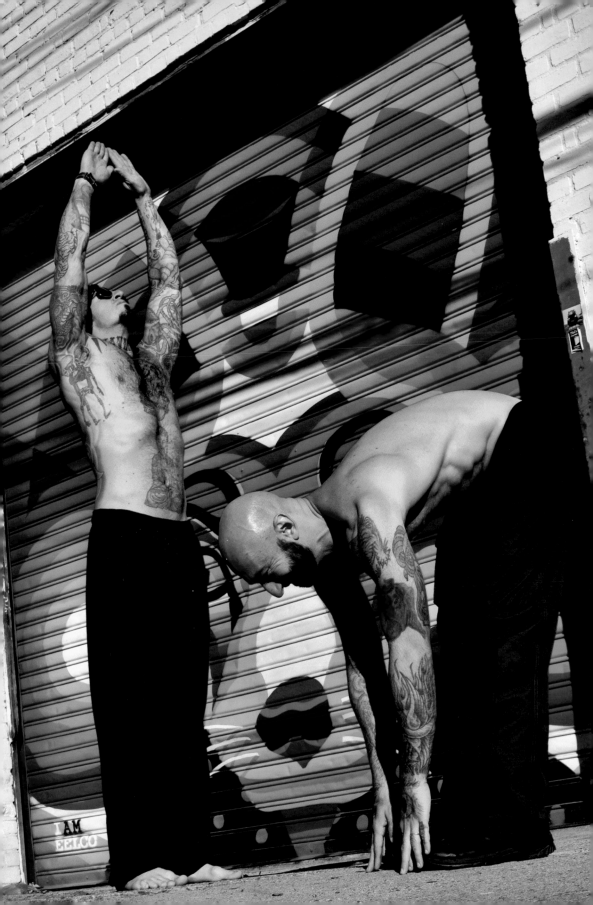

THE
WARM-UP

Preparing your joints, muscles and connective tissue is an important part of strength training. The following warm-ups also fire up your nervous system in preparation for the workout. That's right—these exercises help prepare both the body and mind for what is to come. They will be performed before every training session and may also be used on rest days for active recovery.

Our five warm-up exercises are: Wrist Roll, Reach and Touch, Downdog/Updog Switch, Hollow Body and Plank. They will get your blood flowing, elevate your heart rate and help you get focused. For each warm-up, we've included a three-step description as well as "Trainer Talk" providing further insight. Also included is a list of the muscles that are primarily emphasized in each movement. Be mindful, however, that all of the warm-ups employ the full body.

Take your time and aim to perform them in sequence for approximately 30 seconds each, with short breaks in between as needed. Don't concern yourself with performing a strict number of reps. Instead, go slowly, focusing on the quality of movement while allowing yourself the time to mentally transition into training mode. The entire warm-up should not require more than five minutes.

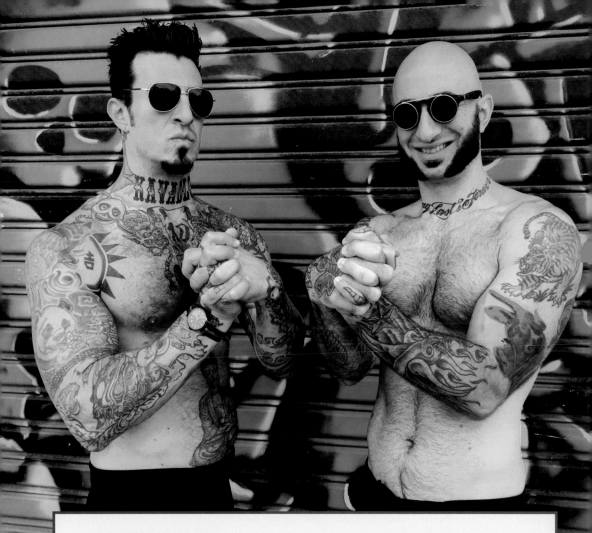

WRIST ROLL

1   Clasp your hands together with your palms facing each other and your fingers interlaced.

2   Keep your arms loose and relaxed as you begin to flex and extend your wrists in a circular motion, rolling your hands up, down, in and out.

3   Reverse the direction and repeat.

Trainer Talk: After several repetitions in both directions, reverse which hand is interlaced on top and repeat.

Muscles Emphasized: Wrists, hands, forearms.

REACH AND TOUCH

1   Stand upright and reach your arms overhead, lengthening your body as much as you can.

2   Bend over and reach for your toes, focusing on keeping your legs as straight as possible, though some knee bending may be unavoidable.

3   Return to an upright position and repeat step one.

Trainer Talk: You may find it helpful to inhale as you stretch your arms overhead and exhale as you reach for your toes.

Muscles Emphasized: Shoulders, lats, abs, lower back, hamstrings, calves, wrists.

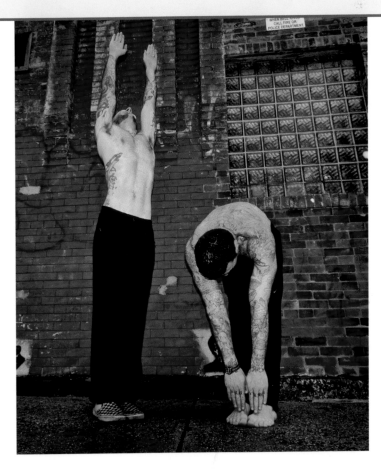

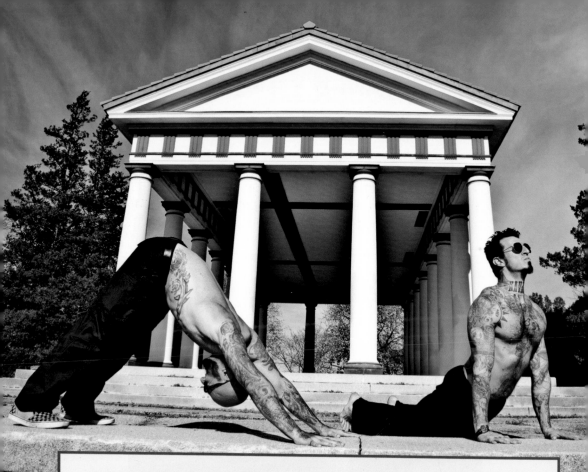

DOWNDOG/UPDOG SWITCH

1   Place your hands and feet on the floor, with your hips raised in the air. Aim to lift your hips as high as possible while keeping your arms and legs as straight as you can manage.

2   Slowly lower your hips and shift your shoulders forward until your chest is above your hands with your hips down by the ground. Maintain straight arms and legs the entire time.

3   Raise your hips into the air and press your chest toward your thighs to return to the start position, again maintaining straight arms and legs the entire time.

Trainer Talk: Take your time in both the top and bottom positions in order to maximize the benefits.

Muscles Emphasized: Shoulders, lats, abs, lower back, hamstrings, calves.

HOLLOW BODY

1   Lie on your back with your legs straight and arms extended overhead. Brace your abs, tuck your chin toward your chest and press your lower back into the ground.

2   Carefully lift your arms and legs, keeping your heels just a few inches from the floor, while maintaining the flat-back (hollow) position.

3   Hold this position, being mindful to avoid any arching in your lower back.

Trainer Talk: If you are unable to perform the full hollow body position, you may try it with your arms at your sides and/or your knees bent.

Muscles Emphasized: Abs, quadriceps, hip flexors.

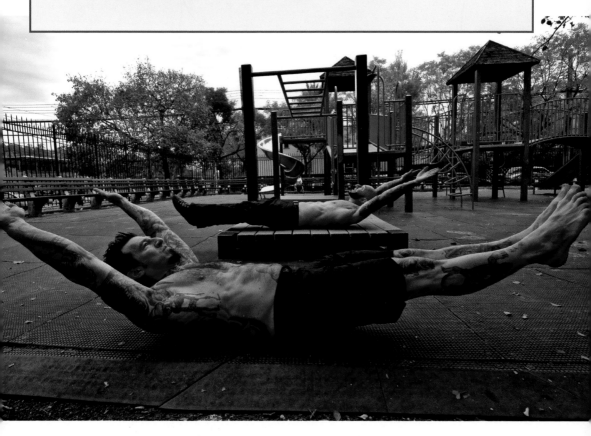

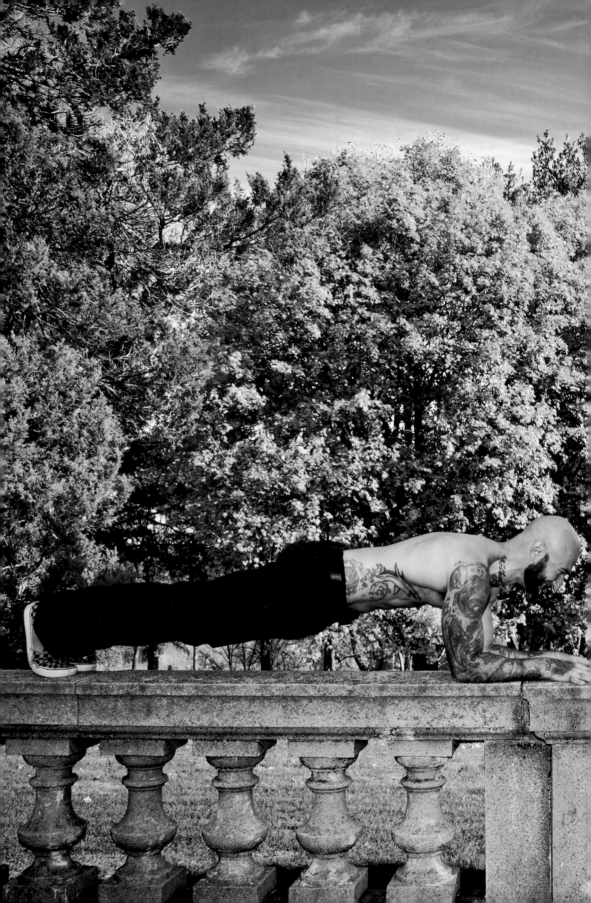

PLANK

1   Place your forearms on the ground parallel to one another, then extend your legs to form a straight line from your heels to the back of your head.

2   Actively pull your shoulder blades down and spread them apart while pressing into the ground with your elbows and forearms. Don't let your shoulders shrug up by your ears.

3   Hold this position, being mindful not to let your hips sag. Watch out that they don't wind up too high in the air either.

Trainer Talk: If you are unable to hold the full plank position, try modifying it by placing your forearms on an elevated surface.

Muscles Emphasized: Shoulders, abs, glutes, lower back.

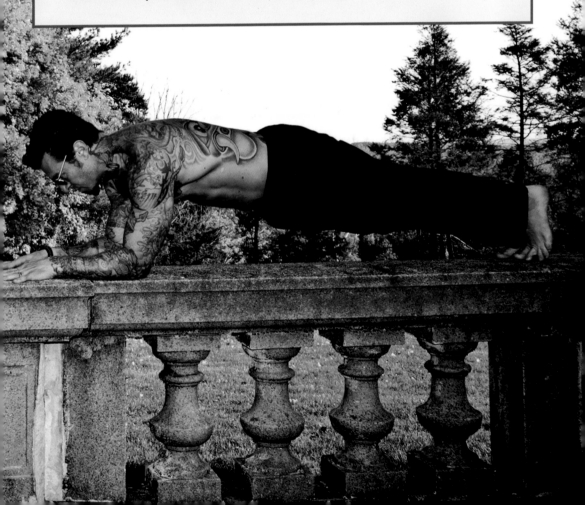

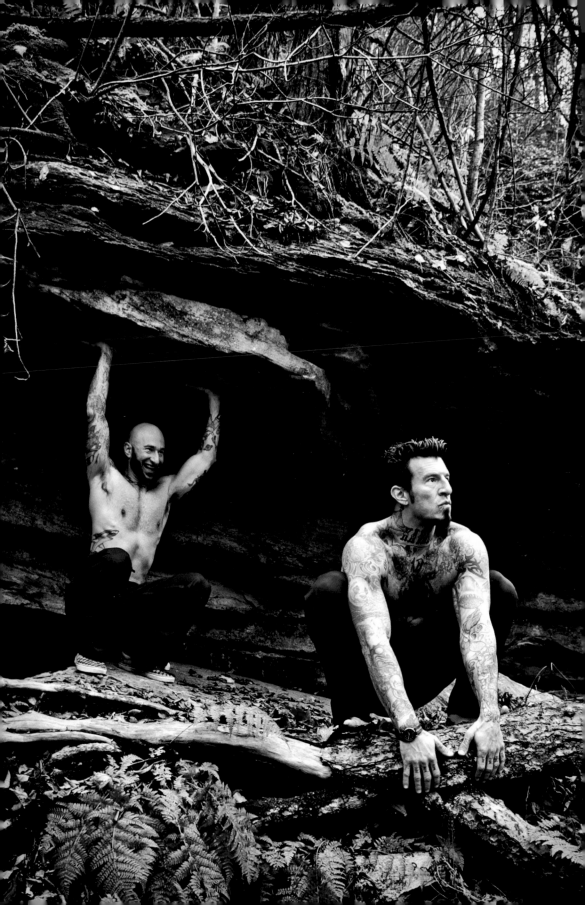

PHASE 1

THE FOUNDATION

This phase is designed to lay a foundation of strength that will allow you to properly progress to more advanced exercises. We will be focusing on six movements during Phase 1: Hands Elevated Push-up, Flex Hang, Active Hang, Lying Knee Tuck, Assisted Squat and Hip Bridge. For each exercise, we've included a three-step description as well as "Trainer Talk" providing further insight. Also included is a list of the muscles that are primarily emphasized in each movement. Be mindful, however, that all of the exercises employ the full body. During each week of this phase, you will be gradually increasing the amount of reps performed on each exercise as your strength and endurance improve.

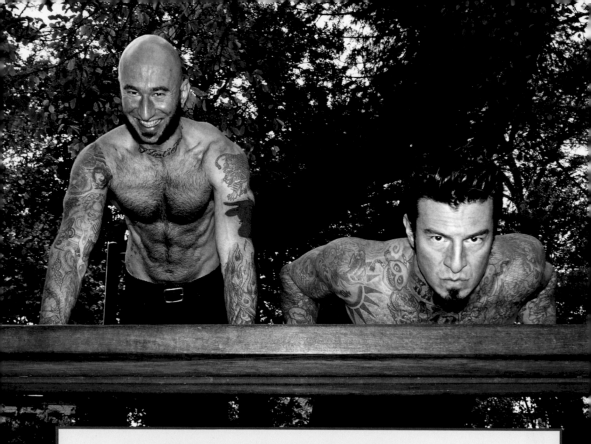

HANDS ELEVATED PUSH-UP

1   Place your hands slightly wider than shoulder width apart on
    an elevated surface of approximately knee height, with your
    feet together and your body in a straight line from your head to
    your heels.

2   Bend your arms and lower your chest toward the elevated sur-
    face, making sure to keep your elbows fairly close to your sides.

3   Pause briefly with your chest approximately one inch from the
    elevated surface, then press yourself back to the top, maintain-
    ing tension in your abs and legs the entire time.

Trainer Talk: If you are unable to perform this exercise on an elevat-
             ed surface of knee height, it may be helpful to use a
             higher surface.

Muscles Emphasized: Chest, shoulders, triceps.

FLEX HANG

1   Stand on an elevated surface in front of a pull-up bar and grab the bar tightly with an underhand grip.

2   With your chin above the bar, hug the bar toward your chest, tense your midsection and carefully step your feet off of the surface, maintaining a flexed-arm position.

3   Hold here, then lower yourself down until your arms are straight before coming off the bar.

Trainer Talk: Lower yourself down from the flex-arm position as slowly as possible. This is sometimes referred to as a "negative" chin-up. It will help you build the strength and control to perform full chin-ups.

Muscles Emphasized: Lats, biceps, abs, grip.

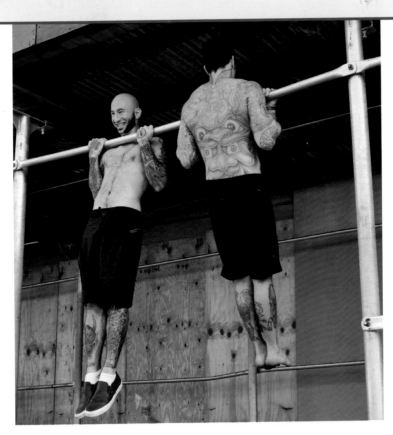

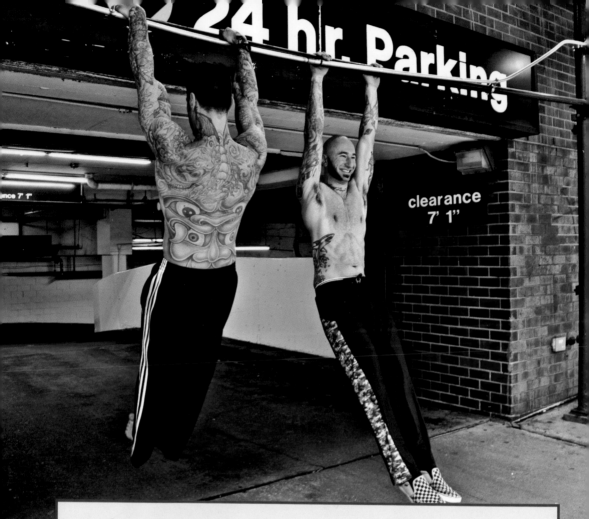

ACTIVE HANG

1   *Grasp an overhead bar with an overhand grip.*

2   *Squeeze your shoulder blades down and back as you lift your feet from the floor, keeping your legs slightly in front of your body with your abs braced.*

3   *Hold the position, being mindful to maintain tension throughout your body.*

Trainer Talk: *This position is s[...] except now you [...]*

Muscles Emphasized: *Lats, a[...]*

add:
SEATED DIP
(upstairs tub)
after ACTIVE HANG

LYING KNEE TUCK

1   Lie on your back with your legs extended and hands at your sides. Lift your heels and press your lower back into the ground.

2   Brace your abs and pull your knees toward your chest.

3   Extend your legs back out without letting your heels touch the floor. Make sure to maintain contact between the ground and your lower back the entire time.

Trainer Talk: If you want to make this exercise more challenging, you can increase the range of motion by lifting your hips off the ground as your knees come toward your chest.

Muscles Emphasized: Abs, hip flexors.

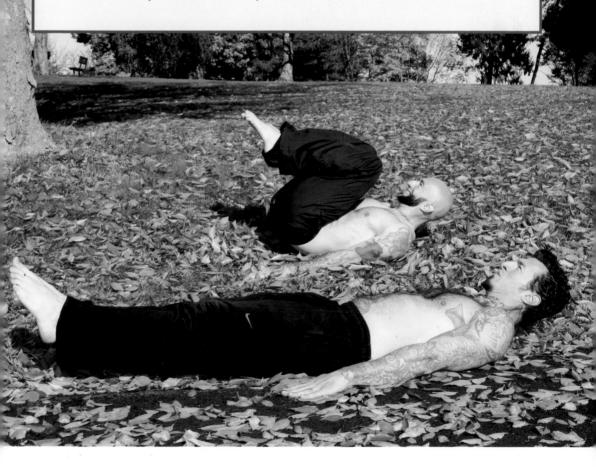

ASSISTED SQUAT

1   Stand up straight with your back toward an elevated surface of
    approximately knee height.

2   Reach your arms forward and bend from your hips, knees and
    ankles, as you carefully sit back onto the elevated surface, mak-
    ing sure to keep your heels flat on the ground the entire time.

3   Pause briefly at the bottom before standing back up to the top
    position.

Trainer Talk: If you are unable to perform this exercise on an elevated surface of knee height, it may be helpful to use a
higher surface.

Muscles Emphasized: Quadriceps, hamstrings, glutes,
calves, lower back.

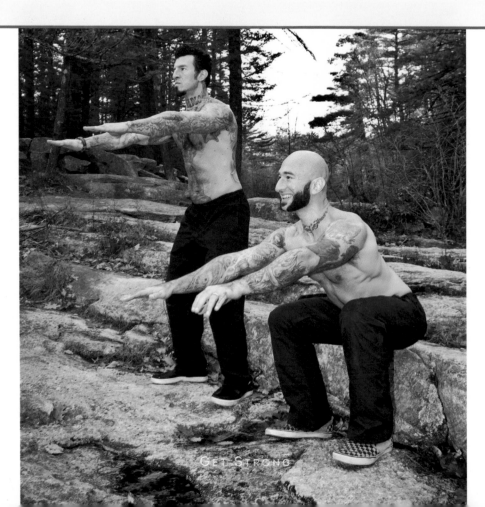

GET STRONG

HIP BRIDGE

1   Lie on the ground face up with your hands by your sides and your knees bent so that your feet are flat on the floor.

2   Press your heels into the ground, lifting your hips as high as you can while creating an arch in your back.

3   Pause briefly before returning to the start position..

Trainer Talk: Focus on squeezing your glutes in order to lift your hips higher.

Muscles Emphasized: Glutes, hamstrings, lower back.

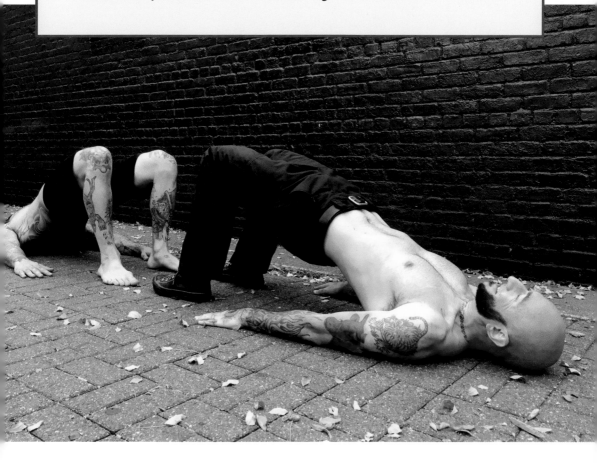

PHASE 1 - WEEK 1

- Repeat this workout three times this week with at least one day off between each session.

- Following the warm-up described earlier, perform all exercises in sequence as written, resting for approximately 60-90 seconds between each set.

- All reps are to be performed with a controlled cadence and full range of motion.

- If you fail to complete the necessary reps, you may add additional sets in order to get them finished.

- Do not move onto Week 2 until you can complete Week 1 as written. If you cannot do so, then repeat Week 1.

Hands Elevated Push-up	3 sets x 6 reps
Flex Hang	3 sets x 5 seconds
Active Hang	3 sets x 10 seconds
Lying Knee Tuck	3 sets x 8 reps
Assisted Squat	3 sets x 10 reps
Hip Bridge	3 sets x 10 reps

PHASE 1 - WEEK 2

- Repeat this workout three times this week with at least one day off between each session.

- Following the warm-up described earlier, perform all exercises in sequence as written, resting for approximately 60-90 seconds between each set.

- All reps are to be performed with a controlled cadence and full range of motion.

- If you fail to complete the necessary reps, you may add additional sets in order to get them finished.

- Do not move onto Week 3 until you can complete Week 2 as written. If you cannot do so, then repeat Week 2.

Hands Elevated Push-up	3 sets x 8 reps
Flex Hang	3 sets x 10 seconds
Active Hang	3 sets x 20 seconds
Lying Knee Tuck	3 sets x 10 reps
Assisted Squat	3 sets x 12 reps
Hip Bridge	3 sets x 12 reps

Phase 1 - Week 3

- Repeat this workout three times this week with at least one day off between each session.

- Following the warm-up described earlier, perform all exercises in sequence as written, resting for approximately 60-90 seconds between each set.

- All reps are to be performed with a controlled cadence and full range of motion.

- If you fail to complete the necessary reps, you may add additional sets in order to get them finished.

- Do not move onto Week 4 until you can complete Week 3 as written. If you cannot do so, then repeat Week 3.

Hands Elevated Push-up	3 sets x 10 reps
Flex Hang	3 sets x 15 seconds
Active Hang	3 sets x 30 seconds
Lying Knee Tuck	3 sets x 12 reps
Assisted Squat	3 sets x 15 reps
Hip Bridge	3 sets x 15 reps

Phase 1 - Week 4

- Repeat this workout three times this week with at least one day off between each session.

- Following the warm-up described earlier, perform all exercises in sequence as written, resting for approximately 60-90 seconds between each set.

- All reps are to be performed with a controlled cadence and full range of motion.

- If you fail to complete the necessary reps, you may add additional sets in order to get them finished.

- At the end of week 4, take the Phase 1 Test to assess if you are ready to advance to Phase 2.

Hands Elevated Push-up	3 sets x 15 reps
Flex Hang	3 sets x 20 seconds
Active Hang	3 sets x 40 seconds
Lying Knee Tuck	3 sets x 15 reps
Assisted Squat	3 sets x 20 reps
Hip Bridge	3 sets x 20 reps

Phase 1
Test Yourself!

If you can complete the following workout in sequence with less than 60 seconds between each exercise, then move onto Phase 2 the following week. If you cannot complete the test as follows, repeat weeks 3 and 4. Test yourself again in two weeks' time.

You may choose to do the test in place of your third training day of week 4 or you may do it as the first day of the following week. Either way, give yourself two full days off from any formal strength training before attempting this test.

TAKE TWO FULL DAYS REST BEFORE THIS TEST

✔ Hands Elevated Push-up .... 1 set x 30 reps

✔ Flex Hang.. 1 set x 30 seconds

✔ Active Hang.. 1 set x 60 seconds

✔ Lying Knee Tuck .... 1 set x 20 reps

✔ Assisted Squat .... 1 set x 30 reps

✔ Hip Bridge... 1 set x 30 reps

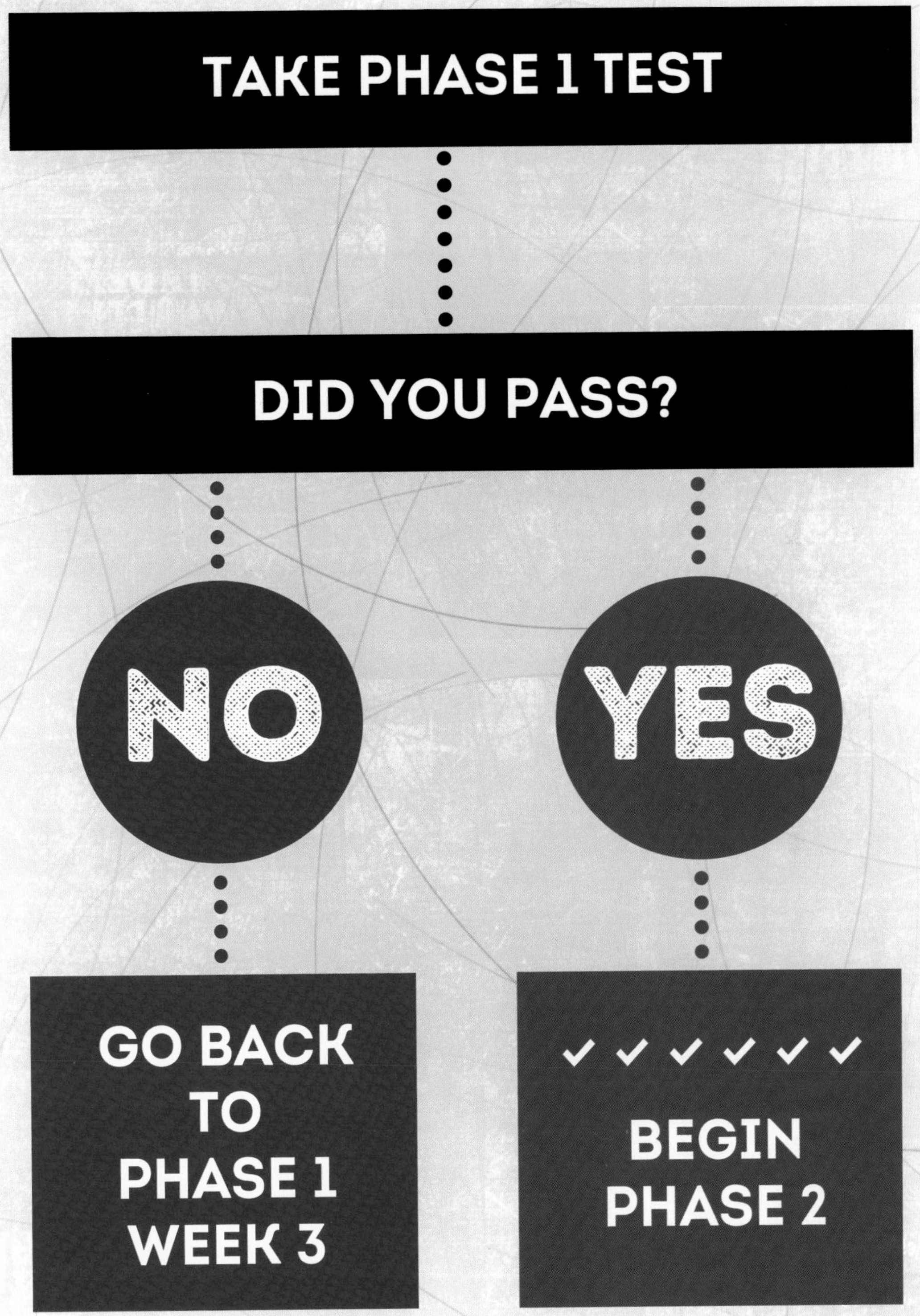

TAKE PHASE 1 TEST

DID YOU PASS?

NO

YES

GO BACK TO PHASE 1 WEEK 3

✓ ✓ ✓ ✓ ✓ ✓

BEGIN PHASE 2

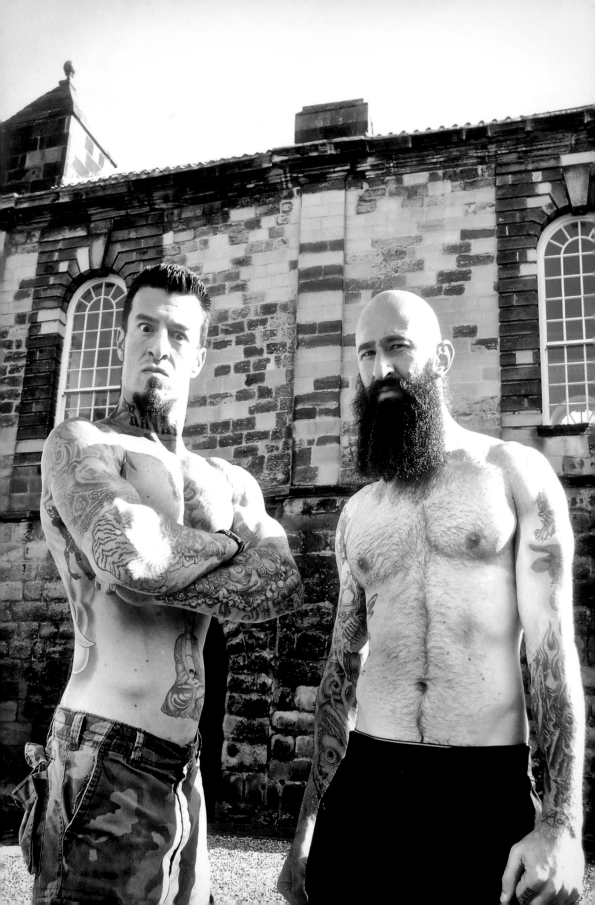

PHASE 2

BRICK AND MORTAR

This phase builds upon your foundation by incorporating the most essential, classic bodyweight strength training exercises. We will be focusing on eight movements during Phase 2: Push-up, Chin-up, Wall Handstand, Hanging Knee Raise, Squat, Split Squat, Step-up and Straight Bridge. For each exercise, we've included a three-step description as well as "Trainer Talk" providing further insight. Also included is a list of the muscles that are primarily emphasized in each movement. Be mindful, however, that all of the exercises employ the full body. You will notice that we are again gradually increasing our reps each week. In some cases, however, we'll be aiming to perform the same number of repetitions in fewer sets. Performing the same workload over fewer sets improves your muscular endurance as you continue to build strength.

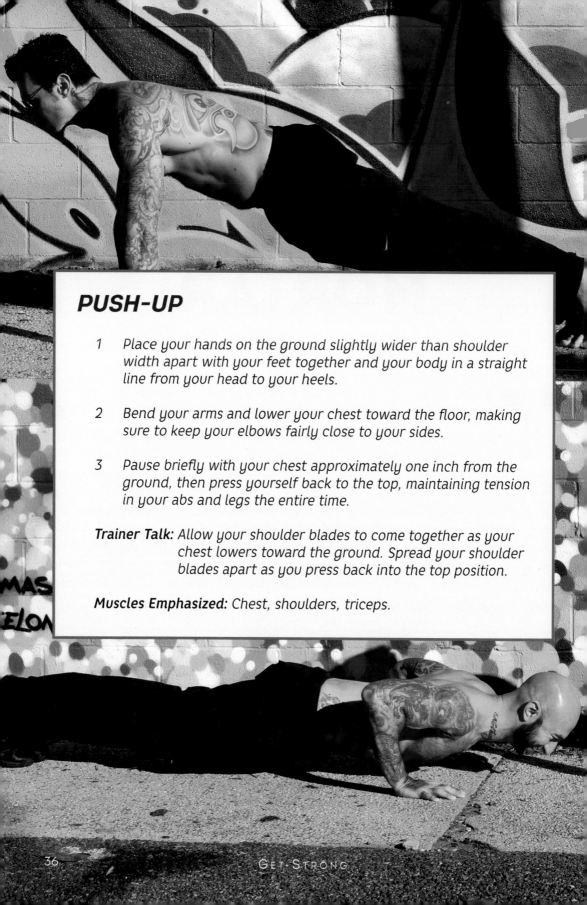

PUSH-UP

1   Place your hands on the ground slightly wider than shoulder width apart with your feet together and your body in a straight line from your head to your heels.

2   Bend your arms and lower your chest toward the floor, making sure to keep your elbows fairly close to your sides.

3   Pause briefly with your chest approximately one inch from the ground, then press yourself back to the top, maintaining tension in your abs and legs the entire time.

Trainer Talk: Allow your shoulder blades to come together as your chest lowers toward the ground. Spread your shoulder blades apart as you press back into the top position.

Muscles Emphasized: Chest, shoulders, triceps.

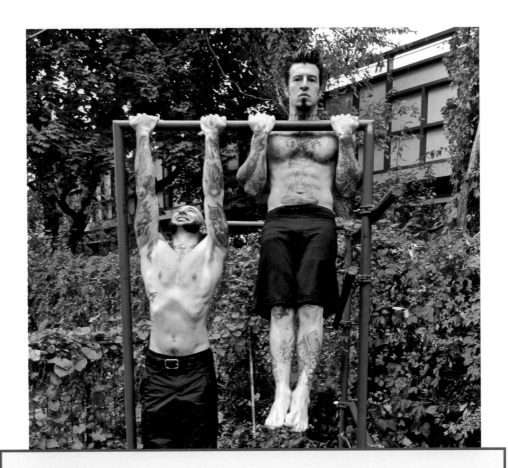

CHIN-UP

1   Begin in the active hang position, except with an underhand grip.

2   Pull yourself up until your chin clears the bar, while maintaining straight legs. Avoid shrugging your shoulders or using any momentum.

3   Lower yourself all the way back to the bottom position with control.

Trainer Talk: *Focus on driving your elbows toward your hips in order to fully engage your lats.*

Muscles Emphasized: *Lats, biceps, abs, grip.*

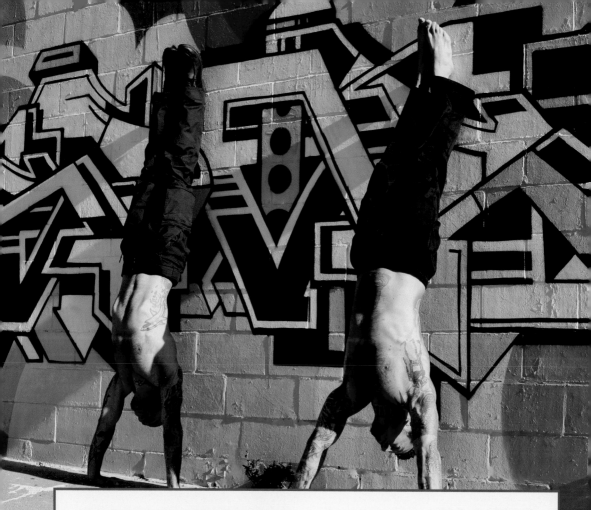

WALL HANDSTAND

1   Place your hands on the floor approximately 6-8 inches away from a wall.

2   Keeping your arms locked, kick your legs into the air until your heels come to rest against the wall.

3   Hold this position for time, being mindful to come down as gently as possible when the set is finished.

Trainer Talk: *Many people will find it helpful to look in between their hands while performing this hold, though others will prefer to keep their head in a neutral position.*

Muscles Emphasized: *Shoulders, chest, triceps, wrists.*

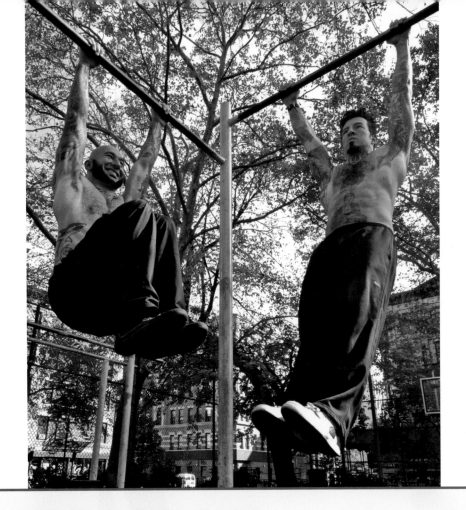

HANGING KNEE RAISE

1   Begin in the active hang position with an overhand grip.

2   Keep your elbows locked and squeeze the bar tightly as you lift
    your knees toward your chest, tilting your pelvis slightly for-
    ward at the top in order to fully engage your abdominals.

3   Lower your legs back to the bottom, being mindful not to swing
    or pick up momentum on the way down.

Trainer Talk: In the bottom position, your feet should be slightly in
front of your body. Do not let your legs swing behind
you.

Muscles Emphasized: Abs, hip flexors, lats, grip.

SQUAT

1   Stand up straight with your feet approximately shoulder width apart.

2   Reach your arms forward and bend from your hips, knees and ankles, lowering until your hamstrings make contact with your calves, while being sure to keep your heels flat on the ground the entire time.

3   Pause briefly at the bottom before standing back up to the top position.

Trainer Talk: Experiment with different foot positions. Some people may feel better with their toes turned out, while others will prefer to keep their feet parallel.

Muscles Emphasized: Quadriceps, hamstrings, glutes, calves, lower back.

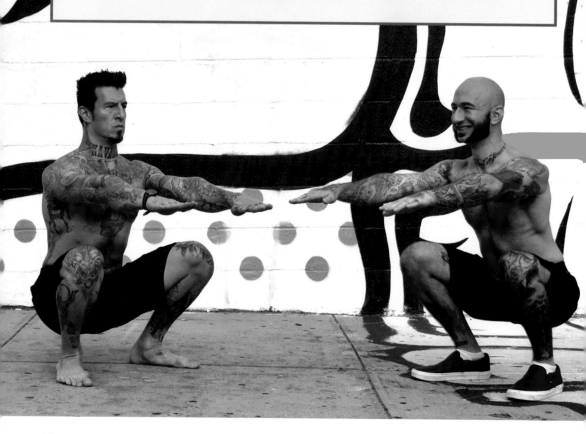

GET STRONG

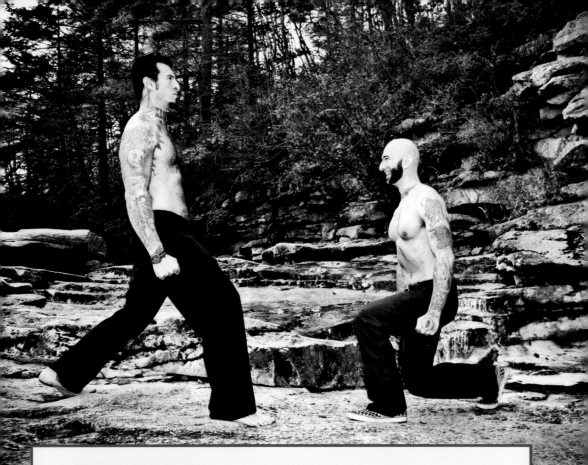

SPLIT SQUAT

1   Stand up straight with your feet approximately shoulder width apart, then take a big step forward with one leg.

2   Keep your torso upright while you lower yourself straight down until both knees are bent to approximately 90 degrees, keeping the front foot totally flat while the back foot comes up onto the toes.

3   Pause briefly at the bottom before standing back up to the top position. Complete your set in its entirety and then repeat on the opposite side.

Trainer Talk: Both legs play a role regardless of which foot is forward. The front foot drives with the heel and the rear foot pushes off with the toes.

Muscles Emphasized: Quadriceps, hamstrings, glutes, calves.

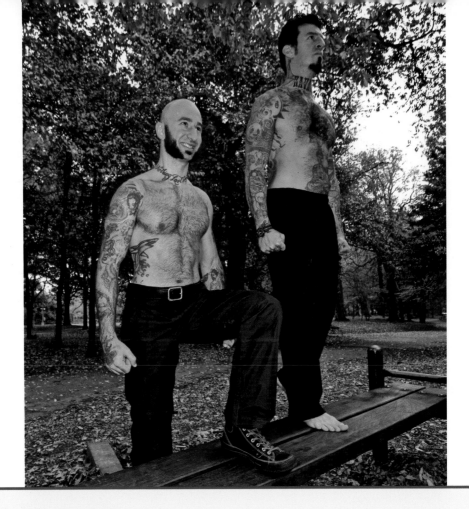

STEP-UP

1   Stand in front of an elevated surface of approximately knee height. Place one foot entirely on the surface.

2   Keep your torso upright while you step up onto the surface, driving with your elevated heel.

3   Keep your foot on the surface and lower your other foot back to the ground. Complete your set in its entirety and then repeat on the opposite side.

Trainer Talk: Focus on using the elevated leg to step up. Avoid relying on the toes of the grounded foot.

Muscles Emphasized: Quadriceps, hamstrings, glutes, calves.

STRAIGHT BRIDGE

1   Sit on the floor with your legs extended straight in front of you
    and your hands just behind your hips.

2   Lift yourself up and straighten out your body by pressing into
    the ground with your hands and heels. Drop your head back,
    press your chest out and look behind you.

3   Pause briefly in the top position, then lower back to the bottom
    with control.

Trainer Talk: Experiment with different hand positions. Some people prefer their fingers pointed forward, while others
feel better with their hands behind them or turned out
to the sides. You can also experiment with pointing or
flexing your toes.

Muscles Emphasized: Glutes, hamstrings, lower back.

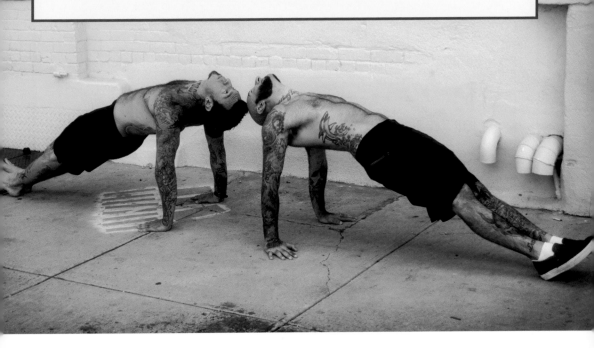

PHASE 2 - WEEK 1

- Repeat this workout three times this week with at least one day off between each session.

- Following the warm-up described earlier, perform all exercises in sequence as written, resting for approximately 60-90 seconds between each set.

- All reps are to be performed with a controlled cadence and full range of motion.

- If you fail to complete the necessary reps, you may add additional sets in order to get them finished.

- Do not move onto Week 2 until you can complete Week 1 as written. If you cannot do so, then repeat Week 1.

Push-up	3 sets x 8 reps
Chin-up	3 sets x 2 reps
Wall Handstand	3 sets x 5 seconds
Hanging Knee Raise	3 sets x 5 reps
Squat	2 sets x 20 reps
Split Squat	2 sets x 10 reps (5 per leg)
Step-up	2 sets x 10 reps (5 per leg)
Straight Bridge	3 sets x 5 reps

Phase 2 - Week 2

- Repeat this workout three times this week with at least one day off between each session.

- Following the warm-up described earlier, perform all exercises in sequence as written, resting for approximately 60-90 seconds between each set.

- All reps are to be performed with a controlled cadence and full range of motion.

- If you fail to complete the necessary reps, you may add additional sets in order to get them finished.

- Do not move onto Week 3 until you can complete Week 2 as written. If you cannot do so, then repeat Week 2.

Push-up	3 sets x 10 reps
Chin-up	3 sets x 3 reps
Wall Handstand	3 sets x 10 seconds
Hanging Knee Raise	3 sets x 8 reps
Squat	3 sets x 20 reps
Split Squat	2 sets x 20 reps (10 per leg)
Step-up	2 sets x 20 reps (10 per leg)
Straight Bridge	3 sets x 8 reps

PHASE 2 - WEEK 3

- Repeat this workout three times this week with at least one day off between each session.

- Following the warm-up described earlier, perform all exercises in sequence as written, resting for approximately 60-90 seconds between each set.

- All reps are to be performed with a controlled cadence and full range of motion.

- If you fail to complete the necessary reps, you may add additional sets in order to get them finished.

- Do not move onto Week 4 until you can complete Week 3 as written. If you cannot do so, then repeat Week 3.

Push-up	3 sets x 12 reps
Chin-up	2 sets x 5 reps
Wall Handstand	2 sets x 20 seconds
Hanging Knee Raise	2 sets x 12 reps
Squat	2 sets x 30 reps
Split Squat	2 sets x 24 reps (12 per leg)
Step-up	2 sets x 24 reps (12 per leg)
Straight Bridge	2 sets x 12 reps

PHASE 2 - WEEK 4

- Repeat this workout three times this week with at least one day off between each session.

- Following the warm-up described earlier, perform all exercises in sequence as written, resting for approximately 60-90 seconds between each set.

- All reps are to be performed with a controlled cadence and full range of motion.

- If you fail to complete the necessary reps, you may add additional sets in order to get them finished.

- At the end of week 4, take the Phase 2 Test to see if you are ready to advance to Phase 3.

Push-up	2 sets x 20 reps
Chin-up	2 sets x 6 reps
Wall Handstand	2 sets x 30 seconds
Hanging Knee Raise	2 sets x 15 reps
Squat	2 sets x 30 reps
Split Squat	2 sets x 30 reps (15 per leg)
Step-up	2 sets x 30 reps (15 per leg)
Straight Bridge	2 sets x 15 reps

PHASE 2
TEST YOURSELF!

If you can complete the following workout in sequence with less than 60 seconds between each exercise, then move onto Phase 3 the following week. If you cannot complete the test as follows, repeat weeks 3 and 4. Test yourself again in two weeks' time.

You may choose to do the test in place of your third training day of week 4 or you may do it as the first day of the following week. Either way, make sure you give yourself two full days off from any formal strength training before attempting this test.

TAKE TWO FULL DAYS REST BEFORE THIS TEST

✔	Push-up	1 set x 30 reps
✔	Chin-up	1 set x 10 reps
✔	Wall Handstand	1 set x 60 seconds
✔	Hanging Knee Raise	1 set x 20 reps
✔	Squat	1 set x 40 reps
✔	Split Squat	1 set x 40 reps (20 per leg)
✔	Step-up	1 set x 40 reps (20 per leg)
✔	Straight Bridge	1 set x 20 reps

TAKE PHASE 2 TEST

DID YOU PASS?

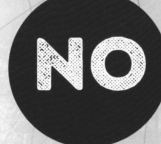

NO

YES

GO BACK TO PHASE 2 WEEK 3

✓ ✓ ✓ ✓ ✓ ✓

BEGIN PHASE 3

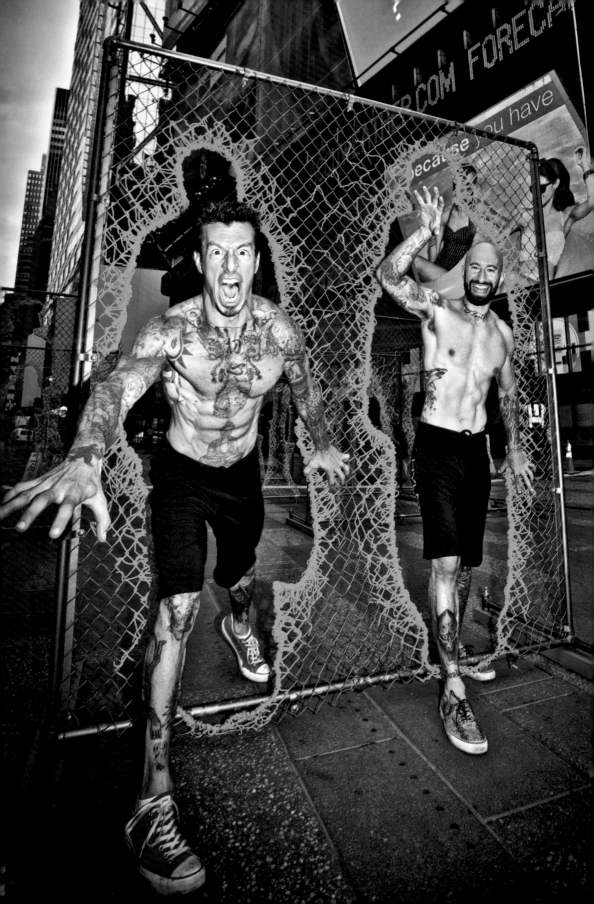

PHASE 3

CONCRETE AND IRON

This phase progresses the classic exercises to the next level and introduces the concept of the split routine. We will no longer be doing three full body workouts each week, instead splitting the training up into two days of upper-body emphasis and two days of lower-body emphasis. This is also the first phase in which we'll be employing single leg exercises.

We will still be using some of the exercises from Phase 2, as well as incorporating eight new movements during Phase 3: Feet Elevated Push-up, Pull-up, Feet Elevated Pike Push-Up, Hanging Straight Leg Raise, Assisted One Leg Squat, Drinking Bird, Bulgarian Split Squat and Candlestick Bridge. For each new exercise, we've included a three-step description as well as "Trainer Talk" providing further insight. Also included is a list of the muscles that are primarily emphasized in each movement. Be aware, however, that all of the exercises employ the full body. You will notice that we are again gradually increasing our reps each week. In some cases, however, we'll be aiming to perform the same number of repetitions in fewer sets. Performing the same workload over fewer sets improves your muscular endurance as you continue to build strength.

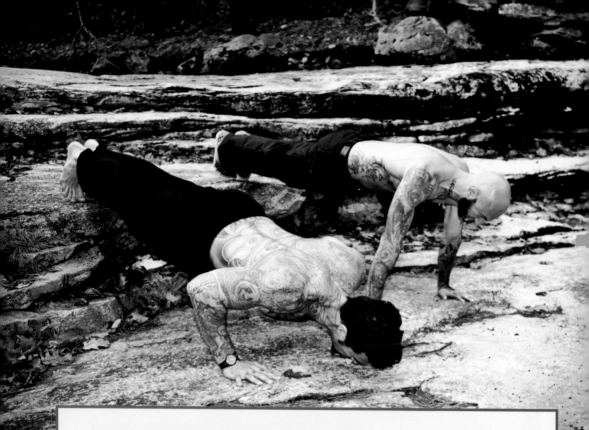

FEET ELEVATED PUSH-UP

1   Place your hands on the ground slightly wider than shoulder
    width apart. Place your feet together on an elevated surface
    of approximately knee height with your body in a straight line
    from your head to your heels.

2   Bend your arms and lower your chest toward the floor, making
    sure to keep your elbows fairly close to your sides.

3   Pause briefly when your nose touches the ground, then press
    yourself back to the top, maintaining tension in your abs and
    legs the entire time.

Trainer Talk: *The height of the surface directly affects how much
weight your arms must bear, with higher surfaces add-
ing increased difficulty. Even a few inches can make a
significant difference.*

Muscles Emphasized: *Chest, shoulders, triceps.*

PULL-UP

1   Begin in the active hang position with an overhand grip.

2   Pull yourself up until your chin clears the bar, while maintaining straight legs. Avoid shrugging your shoulders or using any momentum.

3   Lower yourself back to the bottom position with control.

Trainer Talk: Focus on driving your elbows toward your hips in order to fully engage your lats.

Muscles Emphasized: Lats, biceps, abs, grip.

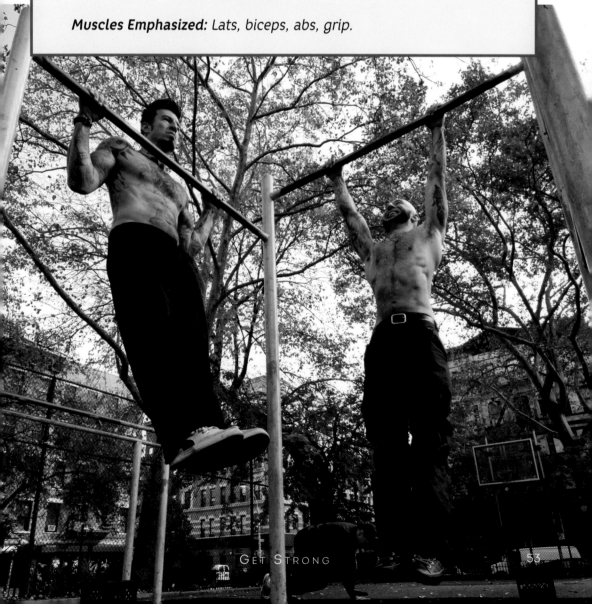

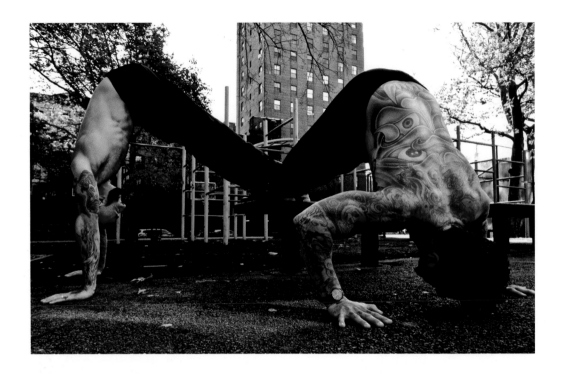

FEET ELEVATED PIKE PUSH-UP

1   Place your hands on the ground slightly wider than shoulder width apart. Place your feet together on an elevated surface of approximately knee height with your hips piked in the air. Your shoulders should be directly beneath your hips.

2   Look in between your hands, bend your arms and lower your head toward the ground.

3   Pause briefly when your nose touches the ground, then press yourself back to the top, making sure to keep your hips directly above your shoulders the whole time.

Trainer Talk: You may feel a deep stretch in your hamstrings during this exercise. Do your best to maintain straight legs.

Muscles Emphasized: Shoulders, chest, triceps, wrists.

HANGING STRAIGHT LEG RAISE

1   Begin in the active hang position with an overhand grip.

2   Keep your knees and elbows locked as you lift your legs up, tilting your pelvis slightly forward, until your legs are parallel to the ground. Flex your quadriceps in order to maintain straight legs.

3   Lower your legs back to the bottom, being mindful not to swing or pick up momentum on the way down.

Trainer Talk:
In the bottom position, your feet should be slightly in front of your body. Do not let your legs swing behind you.

Muscles Emphasized:
Abs, hip flexors, lats, grip.

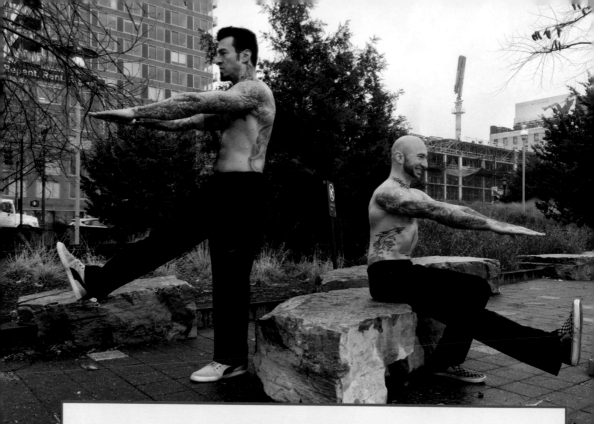

ASSISTED ONE LEG SQUAT

1   Stand up straight with your back toward an elevated surface of
    approximately knee-height, then lift one leg off the ground and
    reach your arms forward.

2   Bend from the hip, knee and ankle of your standing leg to care-
    fully sit back onto the elevated surface, while keeping the other
    leg in the air.

3   Pause briefly at the bottom, then lean forward, drive your heel
    into the ground and brace your trunk to maintain control as you
    stand up. Complete your set in its entirety, then repeat on the
    opposite leg.

Trainer Talk: *If you are unable to perform this exercise on an
elevated surface of knee height, it may be helpful to
use a higher surface.*

Muscles Emphasized: *Quadriceps, hamstrings, glutes, calves, abs,
lower back.*

DRINKING BIRD

1   Stand on one foot with your opposite leg hovering just above the ground behind you.

2   Bend forward at your hips and reach your extended leg behind you, maintaining a straight line from the heel of your extended leg to the back of your head.

3   Pause briefly then return to the start position. Complete your set in its entirety and then repeat on the opposite leg.

Trainer Talk: Be careful not to twist your body to the side when performing this exercise. Focus on keeping your hips even with one another.

Muscles Emphasized: Hamstrings, glutes, calves, lower back.

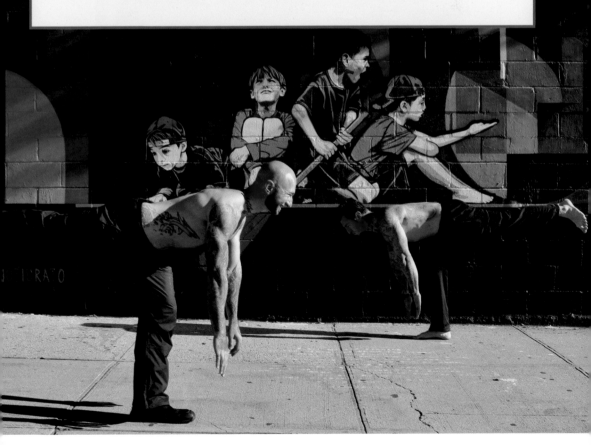

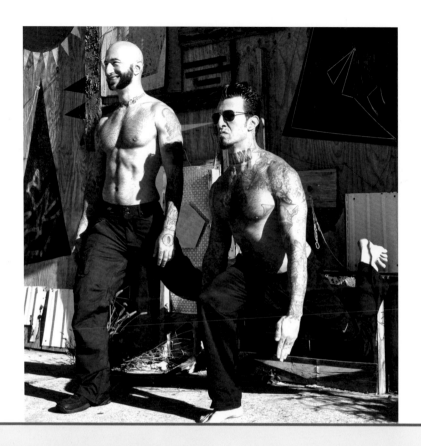

BULGARIAN SPLIT SQUAT

1   *Stand up straight with your back toward an elevated surface of approximately knee height. Lift one foot and place it on the elevated surface behind you.*

2   *Keep your back straight as you lower yourself down until your front knee bends to approximately 90 degrees. Your rear knee will be bent to a more acute angle.*

3   *Pause briefly at the bottom before standing back up to the top position. Complete your set in its entirety and then repeat with your other foot on the elevated surface.*

Trainer Talk: *Keep your front foot totally flat. The rear foot may either come up on the toes or rest on the top of the foot.*

Muscles Emphasized: *Quadriceps, hamstrings, glutes, calves.*

CANDLESTICK BRIDGE

1   Lie on the ground face up with your hands by your sides and your knees bent so your feet are flat on the floor. Raise one leg into the air.

2   Press with your grounded heel, lifting your hips as high as you can while creating an arch with your back.

3   Pause briefly at the top, before returning to the bottom position. Complete your set in its entirety and then repeat on the opposite leg.

Trainer Talk: *Be careful not to twist your body to the side when performing this exercise. Focus on keeping your hips even with one another.*

Muscles Emphasized: *Glutes, hamstrings, lower back.*

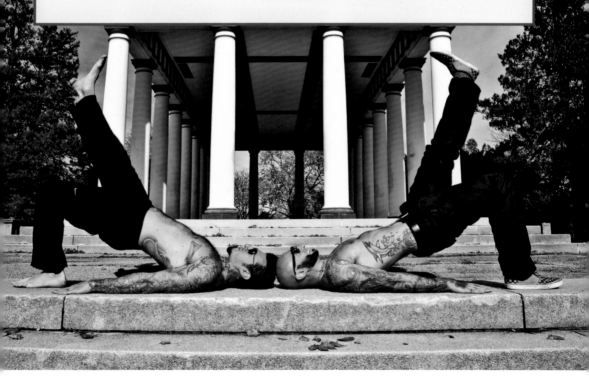

Phase 3 - Week 1

- Repeat each of these workouts twice this week, for a total of four training sessions.

- You may perform the upper body emphasis workout (Workout A) and the lower body emphasis workout (Workout B) on consecutive days, but make sure you have at least 2 days in between repeating the same workout. For example, you may choose to do Workout A on Monday and Thursday, and Workout B on Tuesday and Friday.

- Begin each workout with the warm-up described earlier, then perform all exercises in sequence as written, resting for approximately 60-90 seconds between each set.

- All reps are to be performed with a controlled cadence and full range of motion.

- If you fail to complete the necessary reps, you may add additional sets in order to get them finished. Do not move onto Week 2 until you can complete Week 1 as written. If you cannot do so, then repeat Week 1.

Workout A	Workout B
Feet Elevated Push-up ......3 sets x 10 reps	**Squat** ....2 sets x 20 reps
Pull-up ....2 sets x 5 reps	**Assisted One Leg Squat** ....3 sets x 10 reps (5 per leg)
Feet Elevated Pike Push-up ....3 sets x 5 reps	**Drinking Bird** ....2 sets x 20 reps (10 per leg)
Chin-up ....2 sets x 5 reps	**Bulgarian Split Squat** ....3 sets x 20 reps (10 per leg)
Hanging Straight Leg Raise ....3 sets x 5 reps	**Candlestick Bridge** ....2 sets x 10 reps (5 per leg)
Wall Handstand ....2 sets x 30 seconds	

PHASE 3 - WEEK 2

- Repeat each of these workouts twice this week, for a total of four training sessions.

- You may perform the upper body emphasis workout (Workout A) and the lower body emphasis workout (Workout B) on consecutive days, but make sure you have at least 2 days in between repeating the same workout. For example, you may choose to do Workout A on Monday and Thursday, and Workout B on Tuesday and Friday.

- Begin each workout with the warm-up described earlier, then perform all exercises in sequence as written, resting for approximately 60-90 seconds between each set.

- All reps are to be performed with a controlled cadence and full range of motion.

- If you fail to complete the necessary reps, you may add additional sets in order to get them finished. Do not move onto Week 3 until you can complete Week 2 as written. If you cannot do so, then repeat Week 2.

Workout A	Workout B
Feet Elevated Push-up .....3 sets x 12 reps	Squat ....2 sets x 30 reps
Pull-up ....2 sets x 6 reps	Assisted One Leg Squat ....3 sets x 16 reps (8 per leg)
Feet Elevated Pike Push-up ....3 sets x 6 reps	Drinking Bird ....2 sets x 24 reps (12 per leg)
Chin-up ....2 sets x 6 reps	Bulgarian Split Squat ....3 sets x 24 reps (12 per leg)
Hanging Straight Leg Raise ....3 sets x 6 reps	Candlestick Bridge ....2 sets x 12 reps (6 per leg)
Wall Handstand ....2 sets x 40 seconds	

Phase 3 - Week 3

- Repeat each of these workouts twice this week, for a total of four training sessions.

- You may perform the upper body emphasis workout (Workout A) and the lower body emphasis workout (Workout B) on consecutive days, but make sure you have at least 2 days in between repeating the same workout. For example, you may choose to do Workout A on Monday and Thursday, and Workout B on Tuesday and Friday.

- Begin each workout with the warm-up described earlier, then perform all exercises in sequence as written, resting for approximately 60-90 seconds between each set.

- All reps are to be performed with a controlled cadence and full range of motion.

- If you fail to complete the necessary reps, you may add additional sets in order to get them finished. Do not move onto Week 4 until you can complete Week 3 as written. If you cannot do so, then repeat Week 3.

Workout A	Workout B
Feet Elevated Push-up .....3 sets x 15 reps	Squat ....2 sets x 35 reps
Pull-up ....2 sets x 8 reps	Assisted One Leg Squat ....3 sets x 20 reps (10 per leg)
Feet Elevated Pike Push-up ....3 sets x 8 reps	Drinking Bird ....2 sets x 30 reps (15 per leg)
Chin-up ....2 sets x 8 reps	Bulgarian Split Squat ....3 sets x 24 reps (12 per leg)
Hanging Straight Leg Raise ....3 sets x 8 reps	Candlestick Bridge ....2 sets x 16 reps (8 per leg)
Wall Handstand ....2 sets x 50 seconds	

PHASE 3 - WEEK 4

- Repeat each of these workouts twice this week, for a total of four training sessions.

- You may perform the upper body emphasis workout (Workout A) and the lower body emphasis workout (Workout B) on consecutive days, but make sure you have at least 2 days in between repeating the same workout. For example, you may choose to do Workout A on Monday and Thursday, and Workout B on Tuesday and Friday.

- Begin each workout with the warm-up described earlier, then perform all exercises in sequence as written, resting for approximately 60-90 seconds between each set.

- All reps are to be performed with a controlled cadence and full range of motion.

- If you fail to complete the necessary reps, you may add additional sets in order to get them finished. At the end of week 4, take the Phase 3 Test to see if you are ready to advance to Phase 4.

Workout A		Workout B	
Feet Elevated Push-up	3 sets x 20 reps	Squat	2 sets x 40 reps
Pull-up	2 sets x 10 reps	Assisted One Leg Squat	3 sets x 24 reps (12 per leg)
Feet Elevated Pike Push-up	3 sets x 10 reps	Drinking Bird	2 sets x 30 reps (15 per leg)
Chin-up	2 sets x 10 reps	Bulgarian Split Squat	3 sets x 30 reps (15 per leg)
Hanging Straight Leg Raise	3 sets x 10 reps	Candlestick Bridge	2 sets x 20 reps (10 per leg)
Wall Handstand	2 sets x 60 seconds		

PHASE 3
TEST YOURSELF!

If you can complete the following workout in sequence with less than 60 seconds between each exercise, then move onto Phase 4 the following week. Note that you are only being tested on the new exercises from this phase. If you cannot complete the test as follows, repeat weeks 3 and 4. Test yourself again in two weeks' time.

TAKE TWO FULL DAYS REST BEFORE THIS TEST

- ✔ Feet Elevated Push-up .... 1 set x 30 reps

- ✔ Pull-up .... 1 set x 15 reps

- ✔ Feet Elevated Pike Push-up .... 1 set x 15 reps

- ✔ Hanging Straight Leg Raise .... 1 set x 15 reps

- ✔ Assisted One Leg Squat .... 1 set x 30 reps (15 per leg)

- ✔ Drinking Bird .... 1 set x 40 reps (20 per leg)

- ✔ Bulgarian Split Squat .... 1 set x 40 reps (20 per leg)

- ✔ Candlestick Bridge .... 1 set x 30 reps (15 per leg)

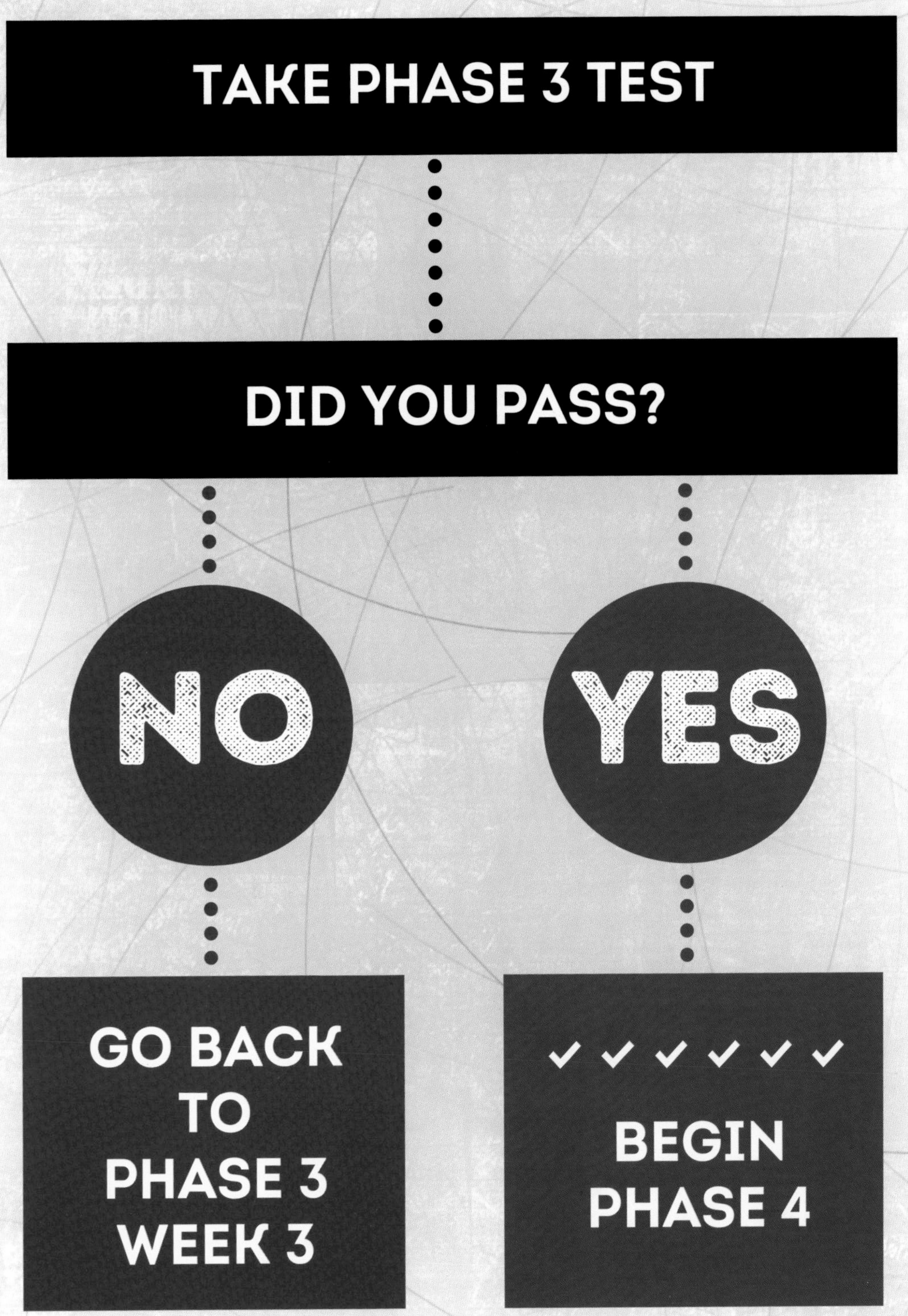

TAKE PHASE 3 TEST

DID YOU PASS?

NO

YES

GO BACK
TO
PHASE 3
WEEK 3

✔ ✔ ✔ ✔ ✔ ✔

BEGIN
PHASE 4

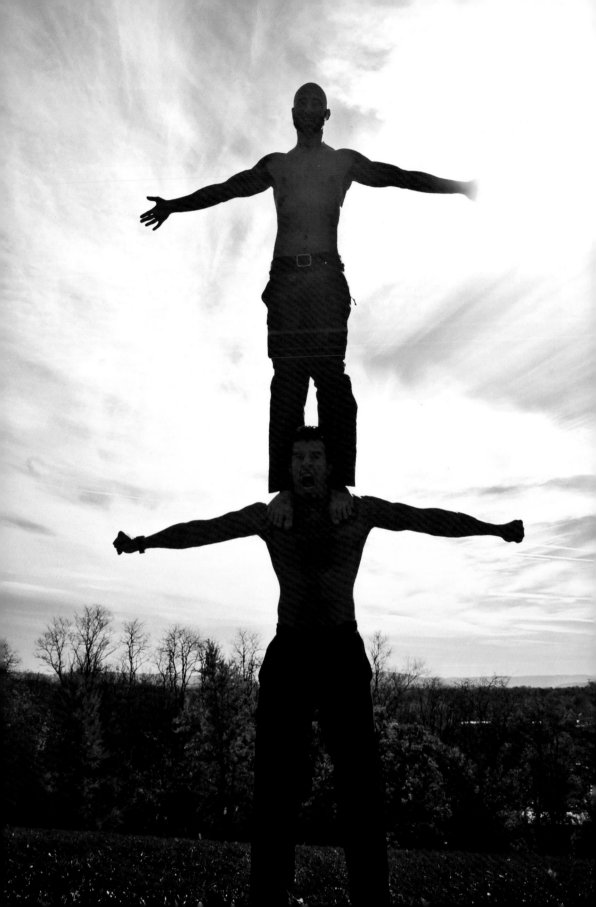

PHASE 4

FORGED FROM STEEL

By this point, you have already gotten results. Phase 4 consists of more advanced exercises designed to push your limits to the edge. This phase introduces more single leg variants, as well as several unilateral moves, where opposing limbs perform different roles.

We will still be using some of the exercises from Phase 2 and Phase 3, as well as incorporating eight new movements during Phase 4: Archer Push-up, Archer Pull-up, Handstand Push-up, Toes to Bar Leg Raise, Archer Squat, Hover Lunge, One Leg Squat and Candlestick Straight Bridge. For each exercise, we've included a three-step description as well as "Trainer Talk" providing further insight. Also included is a list of the muscles that are primarily emphasized in each movement. Be aware, however, that all of the exercises employ the full body.

We will once again be progressively increasing the intensity of the training with each subsequent week. You may notice that the increase in training volume is more gradual in this phase. As one grows stronger, more time and effort are required to continue moving ahead.

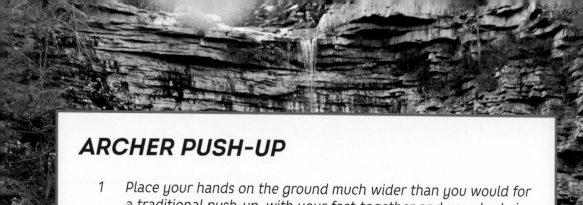

ARCHER PUSH-UP

1   Place your hands on the ground much wider than you would for a traditional push-up, with your feet together and your body in a straight line from your head to your heels.

2   Bend one arm and lower your chest toward the floor on that side. Keep your other arm straight and allow that hand to pivot on the ground.

3   Pause briefly with your chest approximately one inch from the ground, then press yourself back to the top, maintaining tension in your abs and legs the entire time to avoid twisting at your hips. Repeat on the opposite side.

Trainer Talk: *If you are unable to perform an archer push-up with your extended arm completely straight, a small kink at the elbow is acceptable.*

Muscles Emphasized: *Chest, shoulders, triceps.*

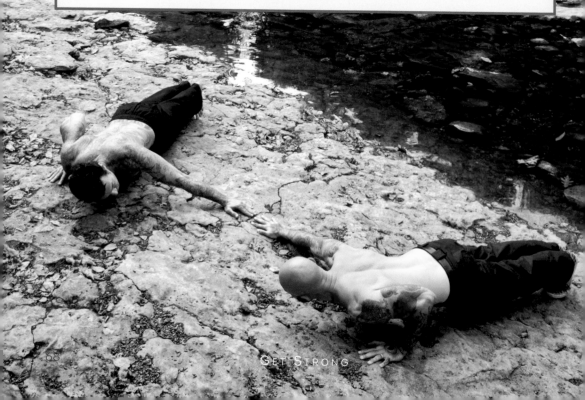

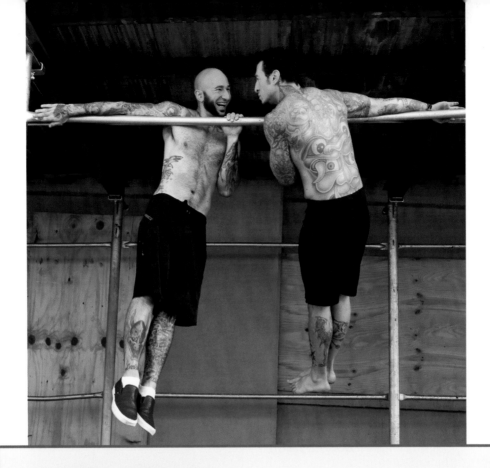

ARCHER PULL-UP

1   Begin in the active hang position with an overhand grip, positioning your hands much wider than you would for a traditional pull-up.

2   Pull yourself up and to the side, bending only at one arm, while keeping your other arm as straight as possible, until your chin clears the bar. Maintain straight legs and avoid shrugging your shoulders or using any momentum.

3   Lower back to the bottom position with control and repeat on the opposite side.

Trainer Talk: Allow the hand of the extended arm to rotate around the bar in order to help facilitate a full range of motion.

Muscles Emphasized: Lats, biceps, abs, grip.

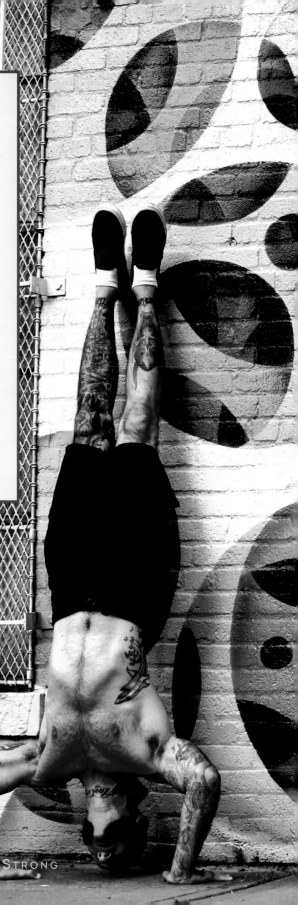

HANDSTAND PUSH-UP

1 Place your hands on the floor approximately 6-8 inches away from a wall. Keeping your arms locked, kick your legs into the air until your heels come to rest against the wall.

2 Look in between your hands, bend your arms and lower your head toward the ground.

3 Pause briefly when your nose touches the floor, then press yourself back to the top, maintaining full body tension the entire time.

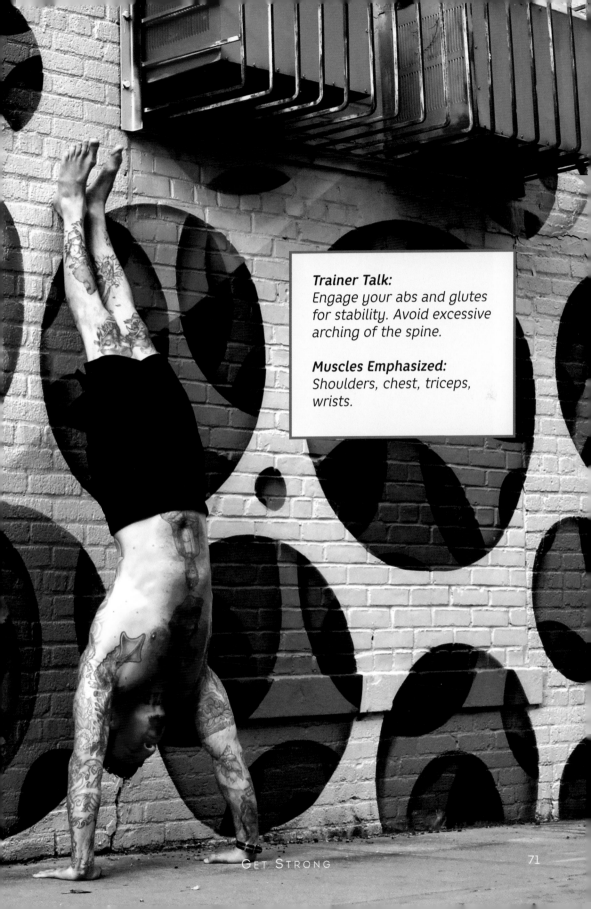

Trainer Talk:
Engage your abs and glutes for stability. Avoid excessive arching of the spine.

Muscles Emphasized:
Shoulders, chest, triceps, wrists.

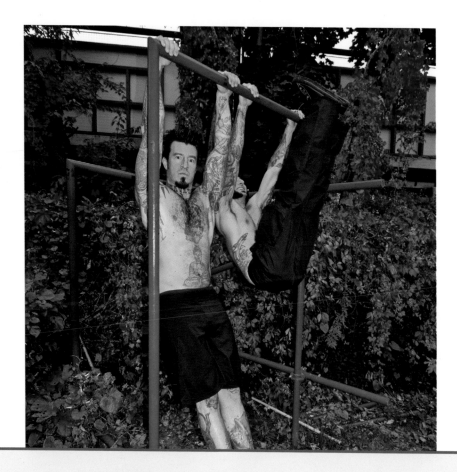

TOES TO BAR LEG RAISE

1   *Begin in the active hang position with an overhand grip.*

2   *Keep your knees and elbows locked and squeeze the bar tightly as you lift your legs up, tilting your pelvis slightly forward. Continue until your toes come in contact with the bar. Flex your quadriceps in order to maintain straight legs.*

3   *Return to the active hang position, being mindful not to swing or pick up momentum on the way down.*

Trainer Talk: *In addition to raising your legs, it can be helpful to envision driving the bar down toward your toes.*

Muscles Emphasized: *Abs, hip flexors, lats, grip.*

ARCHER SQUAT

1   Stand up straight in an extra wide stance with your toes
    pointed out at approximately 45 degrees.

2   Shift your weight toward one side and begin squatting with
    that leg, while keeping your other leg straight. Descend until
    your hamstrings make contact with your calf.

3   Pause briefly at the bottom before standing back up to the top
    position. Repeat on the opposite side.

Trainer Talk: Be sure to keep the foot of your squatting leg flat on
the ground the entire time. Allow the other foot to
pivot into a toes-up position.

Muscles Emphasized: Quadriceps, hamstrings, glutes, calves,
lower back, inner thighs.

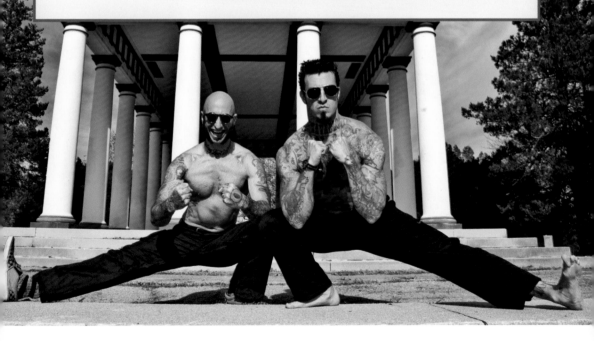

HOVER LUNGE

1   Stand on one foot with your opposite leg bent at the knee and hovering behind you.

2   Reach your arms out, lean forward and bend at the knee, hip and ankle of your standing leg, lowering your opposite knee toward the ground.

3   Pause briefly with your knee approximately one inch from the ground, then return to the top position, maintaining tension in your abs the whole time. Complete your set in its entirety and then repeat on the opposite leg.

Trainer Talk: Descend slowly in order to avoid any potential impact on your rear knee. Make sure the heel of your grounded foot remains flat.

Muscles Emphasized: Quadriceps, hamstrings, glutes, calves, lower back.

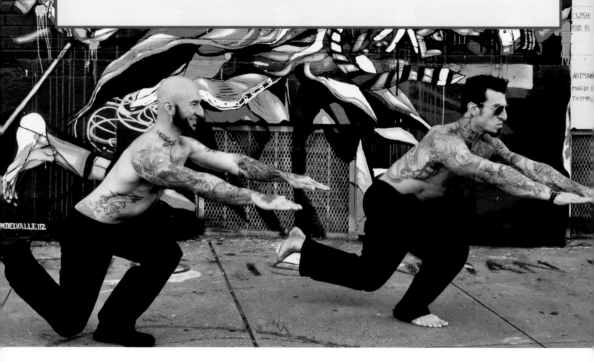

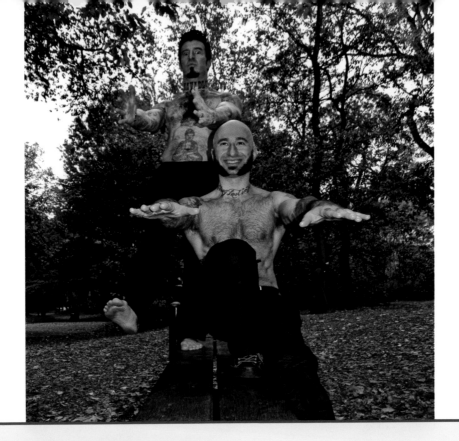

ONE LEG SQUAT

1   Stand on one foot on an elevated surface, with your opposite leg hanging off to the side.

2   Reach your arms forward, as you squat with your standing leg, until your hamstrings make contact with your calf. Be sure to keep that foot flat the entire time. Allow your opposite leg to drop below the elevated surface.

3   Pause briefly at the bottom before standing back up to the top position. Complete your set in its entirety and then repeat on the opposite leg.

Trainer Talk: Think of this exercise like an exaggerated step-up. It has a much greater range of motion and the secondary leg never touches the floor.

Muscles Emphasized: Quadriceps, hamstrings, glutes, calves, lower back.

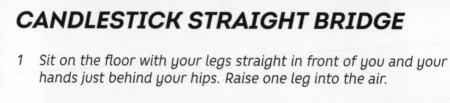

CANDLESTICK STRAIGHT BRIDGE

1   Sit on the floor with your legs straight in front of you and your hands just behind your hips. Raise one leg into the air.

2   Lift yourself up and straighten out your body by pressing into the floor with your hands and grounded heel. Drop your head back, press your chest out and look behind you.

3   Pause briefly in the top position, then lower back to the bottom with control. Complete your set in its entirety and then repeat on the opposite leg.

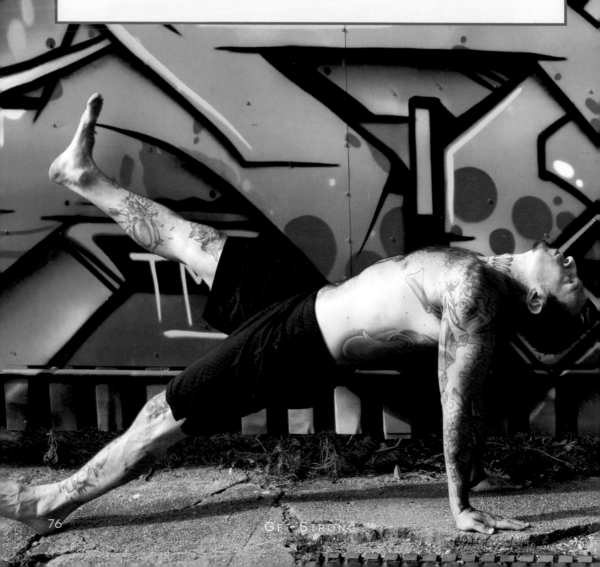

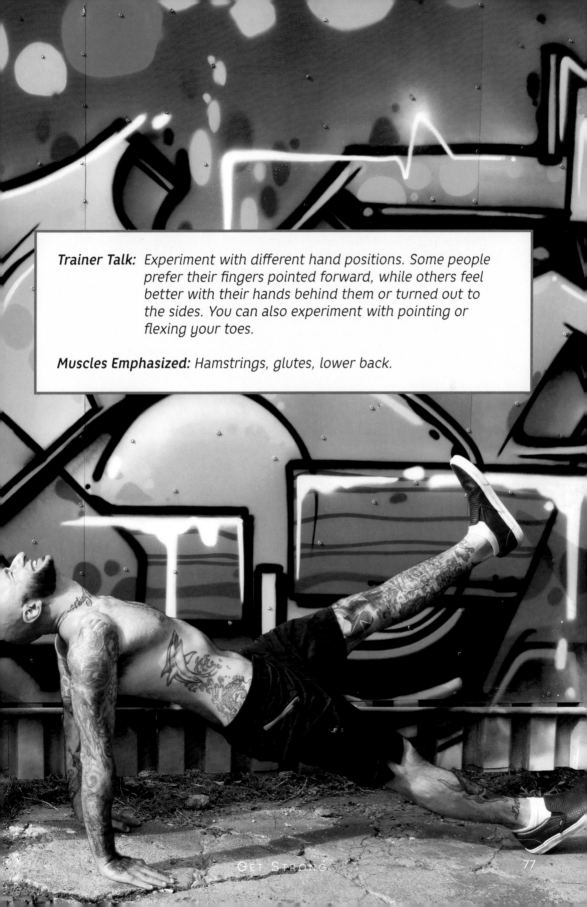

Trainer Talk: *Experiment with different hand positions. Some people prefer their fingers pointed forward, while others feel better with their hands behind them or turned out to the sides. You can also experiment with pointing or flexing your toes.*

Muscles Emphasized: *Hamstrings, glutes, lower back.*

PHASE 4 - WEEK 1

- Repeat each of these workouts twice this week, for a total of four training sessions.

- You may perform the upper body emphasis workout (Workout A) and the lower body emphasis workout (Workout B) on consecutive days, but make sure you have at least 2 days in between repeating the same workout. For example, you may choose to do Workout A on Monday and Thursday, and Workout B on Tuesday and Friday.

- Begin each workout with the warm-up described earlier, then perform all exercises in sequence as written, resting for approximately 60-90 seconds between each set.

- All reps are to be performed with a controlled cadence and full range of motion.

- If you fail to complete the necessary reps, you may add additional sets in order to get them finished. Do not move onto Week 2 until you can complete Week 1 as written. If you cannot do so, then repeat Week 1.

Workout A	Workout B
Feet Elevated Push-up ..... 2 sets x 15 reps	**Squat** ..... 2 sets x 40 reps
Pull-up ..... 2 sets x 8 reps	**Archer Squat** ..... 3 sets x 10 reps (5 per leg)
Archer Push-up ..... 3 sets x 6 reps (3 per side)	**Hover Lunge** ..... 3 sets x 6 reps (3 per leg)
Archer Pull-up ..... 5 sets x 2 reps (1 per side)	**One Leg Squat** ..... 3 sets x 6 reps (3 per leg)
Handstand Push-up ..... 3 sets x 3 reps	**Candlestick Straight Bridge** ..... 2 sets x 10 reps (5 per leg)
Toes to Bar Leg Raise ..... 3 sets x 3 reps	

PHASE 4 - WEEK 2

- Repeat each of these workouts twice this week, for a total of four training sessions.

- You may perform the upper body emphasis workout (Workout A) and the lower body emphasis workout (Workout B) on consecutive days, but make sure you have at least 2 days in between repeating the same workout. For example, you may choose to do Workout A on Monday and Thursday, and Workout B on Tuesday and Friday.

- Begin each workout with the warm-up described earlier, then perform all exercises in sequence as written, resting for approximately 60-90 seconds between each set.

- All reps are to be performed with a controlled cadence and full range of motion.

- If you fail to complete the necessary reps, you may add additional sets in order to get them finished. Do not move onto Week 3 until you can complete Week 2 as written. If you cannot do so, then repeat Week 2.

Workout A

**Feet Elevated
Push-up** .... 2 sets x 20 reps

Pull-up .... 2 sets x 10 reps

Archer Push-up .... 3 sets x 8 reps (4 per side)

Archer Pull-up .... 3 sets x 4 reps (2 per side)

**Handstand
Push-up** .... 2 sets x 5 reps

**Toes to Bar
Leg Raise** .... 2 sets x 5 reps

Workout B

Squat .... 2 sets x 40 reps

Archer Squat .... 3 sets x 12 reps (6 per leg)

Hover Lunge .... 3 sets x 10 reps (5 per leg)

**One Leg
Squat** .... 3 sets x 10 reps (5 per leg)

**Candlestick
Straight Bridge** ...... 2 sets x 12 reps (6 per leg)

PHASE 4 - WEEK 3

- Repeat each of these workouts twice this week, for a total of four training sessions.

- You may perform the upper body emphasis workout (Workout A) and the lower body emphasis workout (Workout B) on consecutive days, but make sure you have at least 2 days in between repeating the same workout. For example, you may choose to do Workout A on Monday and Thursday, and Workout B on Tuesday and Friday.

- Begin each workout with the warm-up described earlier, then perform all exercises in sequence as written, resting for approximately 60-90 seconds between each set.

- All reps are to be performed with a controlled cadence and full range of motion.

- If you fail to complete the necessary reps, you may add additional sets in order to get them finished. Do not move onto Week 4 until you can complete Week 3 as written. If you cannot do so, then repeat Week 3.

Workout A	Workout B
Feet Elevated Push-up ....2 sets x 20 reps	**Squat**........................ 2 sets x 40 reps
Pull-up ....2 sets x 10 reps	**Archer Squat** ....3 sets x 16 reps (8 per leg)
Archer Push-up ....3 sets x 10 reps (5 per side)	**Hover Lunge** ....3 sets x 12 reps (6 per leg)
Archer Pull-up ....4 sets x 4 reps (2 per side)	**One Leg Squat** ....3 sets x 12 reps (6 per leg)
Handstand Push-up ....2 sets x 6 reps	**Candlestick Straight Bridge** .....2 sets x 16 reps (8 per leg)
Toes to Bar Leg Raise ....2 sets x 6 reps	

PHASE 4 - WEEK 4

- Repeat each of these workouts twice this week, for a total of four training sessions.

- You may perform the upper body emphasis workout (Workout A) and the lower body emphasis workout (Workout B) on consecutive days, but make sure you have at least 2 days in between repeating the same workout. For example, you may choose to do Workout A on Monday and Thursday, and Workout B on Tuesday and Friday.

- Begin each workout with the warm-up described earlier, then perform all exercises in sequence as written, resting for approximately 60-90 seconds between each set.

- All reps are to be performed with a controlled cadence and full range of motion.

- If you fail to complete the necessary reps, you may add additional sets in order to get them finished. At the end of week 4, take the Phase 4 Test to see if you have completed the program.

Workout A

Feet Elevated
Push-up ....2 sets x 25 reps

Pull-up ....2 sets x 12 reps

Archer Push-up ....3 sets x 12 reps (6 per side)

Archer Pull-up ....3 sets x 6 reps (3 per side)

Handstand
Push-up ....2 sets x 8 reps

Toes to Bar
 Leg Raise ....2 sets x 8 reps

Workout B

Squat ....2 sets x 50 reps

Archer Squat ....3 sets x 20 reps (10 per leg)

Hover Lunge ....3 sets x 16 reps (8 per leg)

One Leg
Squat ....3 sets x 16 reps (8 per leg)

Candlestick
Straight Bridge ....2 sets x 20 reps (10 per leg)

PHASE 4
TEST YOURSELF!

The following test consists of all the new exercises from this phase. If you can complete the test in sequence with less than 60 seconds between each exercise, then you have completed the *Get Strong* program. Congratulations! You are now officially Kavadlo Brothers Strong!

If you cannot complete the test as follows, repeat weeks 3 and 4. Test yourself again in two weeks' time.

Make sure you give yourself two full days off from any formal strength training before attempting this test.

TAKE TWO FULL DAYS REST BEFORE THIS TEST

- ✔ Archer Push-up ....1 set x 20 reps (10 each side)
- ✔ Archer Pull-up ....1 set x 10 reps (5 each side)
- ✔ Handstand Push-up ....1 set x 10 reps
- ✔ Toes to Bar Leg Raise ....1 set x 10 reps
- ✔ Archer Squat ....1 set x 40 reps (20 each leg)
- ✔ Hover Lunge ....1 set x 20 reps (10 each leg)
- ✔ One Leg Squat ....1 set x 20 reps (10 each leg)
- ✔ Candlestick Straight Bridge ......1 set x 30 reps (15 each leg)

TAKE PHASE 4 TEST

DID YOU PASS?

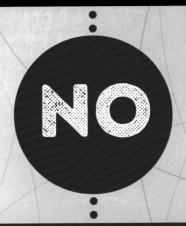

NO

**GO BACK
TO PHASE 4
WEEK 3**

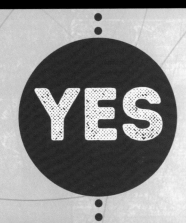

YES

✓ ✓ ✓ ✓ ✓ ✓
**YOU GOT
STRONG!**

You may wind up needing more than 16 weeks to go from the start of Phase 1 to the completion of this program. In all likelihood, you will have setbacks at some point: An illness, injury or unexpected life circumstance may temporarily derail you. This is okay. Just make sure you get back on track as soon as you can. You will learn more from your own trials and errors than from anything else. Enjoy the journey and embrace each step in your progression. With persistence, you will advance in your own time.

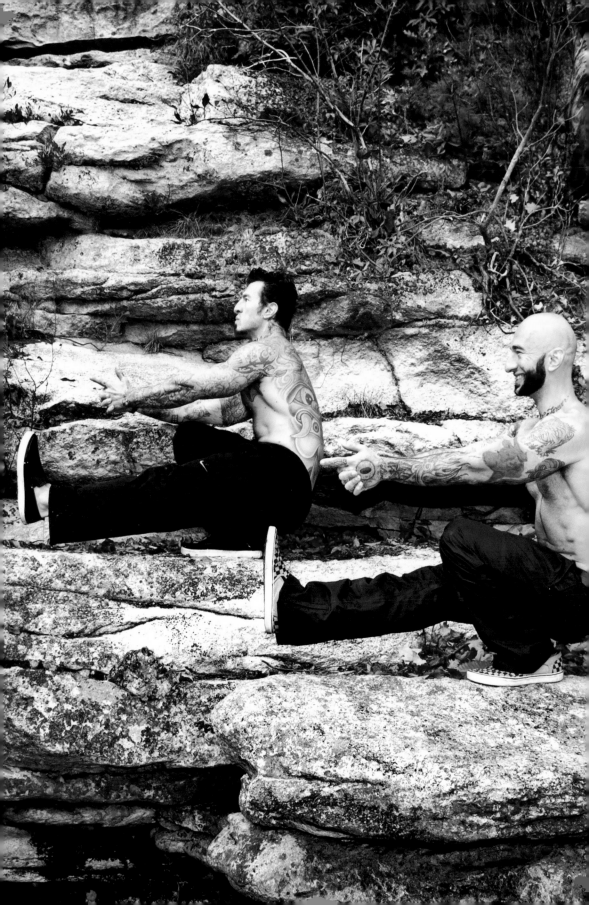

- II -

STAY
STRONG

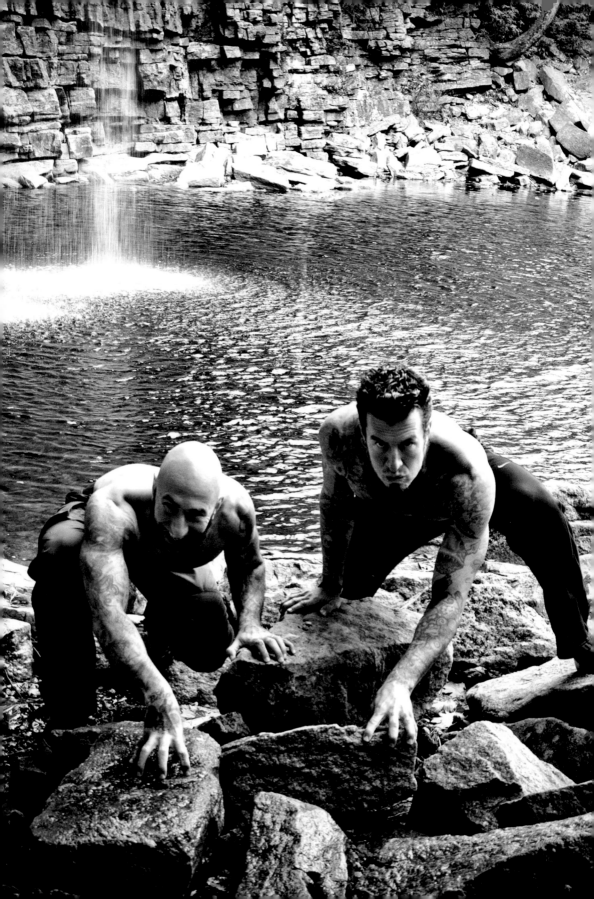

THE END IS THE BEGINNING

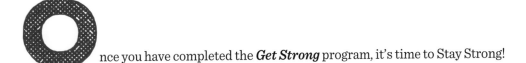nce you have completed the **Get Strong** program, it's time to Stay Strong!

What follows are questions, answers, experience and truth. The words in this section provide actionable advice to help you through your journey and far beyond with confidence, power and grace.

We've also included several supplemental exercises and workouts that are not part of the **Get Strong** program due to equipment requirements or the need for a high prerequisite skill level. As stated earlier, the **Get Strong** program is the most stripped-down, efficient path available. It's the most direct method for building strength and muscle. The exercises and workouts in this section are a fantastic addition.

If you want to delve deeper, check out our book **Street Workout** for dozens more calisthenics progressions.

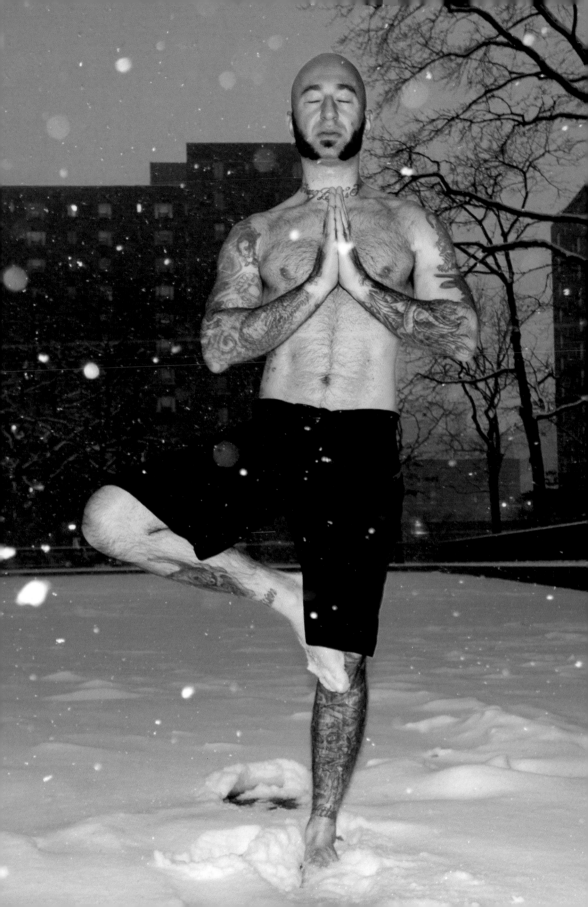

ASK AL

I just started the Get Strong program and I am so sore! Should I still do the prescribed number of training sessions this week or is it okay to do fewer?

Sometimes when you're new to strength training, it can be a shock to the system. After your first workout, it's not unheard of for muscular soreness to linger for an entire week or more, so don't be alarmed if you experience intense soreness at first.

If you need additional rest days, feel free to take them. Furthermore, you may find that during the first week of each phase, you may need additional recovery time due to introducing new movements into your regimen.

I am not even strong enough to do some of the exercises in Phase 1, Week 1 of the Get Strong program. Even some of these warm-ups are hard for me! Am I hopeless? What should I do?

You're not hopeless. In fact, if you stick with your training, you are about to get in the best shape of your life!

There are a few ways you can modify the exercises in Phase 1 to make them more suited to your current strength level. For hands elevated push-ups, you can use a surface that is waist height instead of knee height. You can even use a chest height surface if waist height is still too difficult. You can also use a higher surface for your assisted squats. For flex hangs and active hangs, you can keep one foot on a chair or platform to assist your arms. Put as much of your weight as possible in your arms and use your foot to make up the difference.

As for any other exercises that you cannot perform during Phase 1, you can leave them out for the first 3-4 weeks of your training, then try reincorporating them after you've been consistent for a few weeks. Following this remedial period, you may restart the program on Phase 1, Week 1 as written.

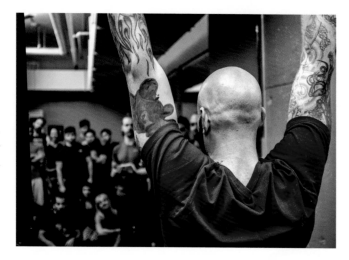

I've been working out for a few years already. Do I have to begin this program at Phase 1 or can I start in at one of the later levels?

If you feel like you are ready to jump in at Phase 2 or Phase 3 of this program, I encourage you to take the Phase 1 test and see how it goes. We often have a tendency to underestimate things when we look at them on paper, but many of these workouts are more difficult than they may appear. Having said that, if you are able to complete the test for a given phase without any issues, then you may begin the program at the following phase.

Why doesn't your program include dips and Aussie pull-ups (bodyweight rows)? Aren't those worthwhile exercises?

Dips and Aussie pull-ups are both fantastic exercises! Danny and I actually went back and forth about whether or not to include them in the **Get Strong** program. Ultimately, we left them out, not because they are useless, but rather because the focus of this program is on exercises that can be done with as little equipment as possible: a pull-up bar, a bench, a wall or the floor. Since dips typically require parallel bars, and Aussie pull-ups require a waist-height bar, we opted to leave them out in favor of more universally available exercises.

Having said that, if you have access to the equipment to do those moves and you want to add them, you have my blessing to incorporate them as you see fit. In fact, they're included in the Supplemental Exercises section in this book. There are lots of great exercises, but not all of them can be in every program.

I've been on the Get Strong program for a couple of months and I'm making good progress. Lately I've found that even though I still feel like I'm training hard, I'm barely sore the day after my workout. Does that mean the training isn't working anymore?

Quite the contrary; not getting sore is a sign that you are getting more fit! When you first started, you would probably feel sore for days following a workout. And it was probably a workout that would barely even get you to break a sweat today. Now you can do intense workouts and your body is able to recover quickly.

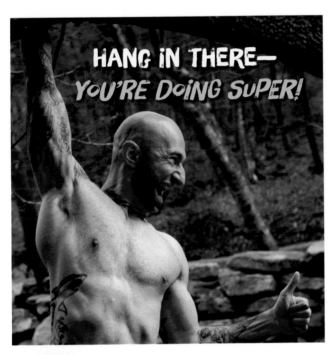

The goal of your training shouldn't be to make you sore; it should be to make you well equipped to handle even the most intense physical conditions without experiencing significant fatigue. It sounds like that's where you're going, so hang in there—you're doing super!

Is it better to train in the morning or at night?

A lot of people like to exercise first thing in the morning in order to get it out of the way. If you do your workout before the stresses of the day start to pile up, then you don't have to worry about life derailing your plans. On the other hand, exercise can be a great way to blow off some steam at the end of the day. Do whatever works best for you. As long as you get your reps in, it doesn't matter.

Overhand pull-ups and underhand chin-ups both kind of hurt my wrists, shoulders and/or elbows. Palms facing each other feels fine, though. Is it OK to just do those, or do I have to stick with the underhand and overhand grips?

Depending on the individual skeletal subtleties of each person's joints, different grips can be more or less favorable for different people. It's not uncommon for fully supinated (underhand) or fully pronated (overhand) grips to impinge the joints in certain individuals. If you feel best working with palms facing each other, then feel free to make that adjustment.

 What about using gymnastic rings for pull-ups?

Sure! Gymnastic rings are unique in that they allow for rotation of your arms throughout the range of motion. Some people find that beginning in a pronated (or partially pronated) position at the bottom of a rep and rotating into a supinated (or partially supinated) position at the top gives them the best of both worlds. I personally feel best with the classic overhand grip on a straight bar, but you've gotta listen to your body and do what's right for you. If you feel better doing your pull-ups on rings, then do so.

 Are squats bad for your knees? I've been doing them for a while but I hear they're bad for your knees.

If you've been doing squats for a while, then you already have firsthand experience from which to draw. If your knees aren't hurting, then there's your answer. Don't let someone else's opinion override your own experience with the world. Having said that, I can tell you from my own experience that squatting has kept my knees strong and supple. I've been doing squats and squat variants as part of my routine for nearly twenty years and my knees feel great. Squats are good for your knees.

However, any exercise is potentially dangerous if it is done with poor form or by a person who is not ready for it, and squats are no exception. As always, your training is what you make of it. If you're sloppy and shortsighted, you may wind up hurting yourself. However, if you approach your training with reverence, you can enjoy the journey for a lifetime.

I can do lots of one leg squats with my left leg, but my right is much weaker, and I struggle to get a few reps. Should I do extra work to make it catch up?

I noticed you said your left leg is stronger than your right—are you right-handed? Though not always the case, it's common for people to be stronger on the leg that's opposite their dominant arm. In many sports and activities, we post off our left leg to use our right hand. Right-handed boxers lead with their left leg, right-handed pitchers throw from their left leg, etc. If you've done these types of contralateral movements (or even if you haven't) there's a good chance you are cross dominant.

So don't worry—it's normal to have some disparity between your two sides. No matter how you train, muscle imbalances are inevitable; the human body is never going to be perfectly symmetrical. However, it's still beneficial to strive for balance between your left and right sides.

I recommend bringing up your less strong leg by prioritizing it in your workouts. For you, this means training your right leg first within each session. This will allow you to give it your full energy and attention. (Someone whose left leg is less strong would train that side first.) You can also spread the same number of reps out over more sets on that side. If the workout calls for 3 sets of 5 reps, you can try doing 5 sets of 3 reps instead in order to allow for more recovery without doing less total work.

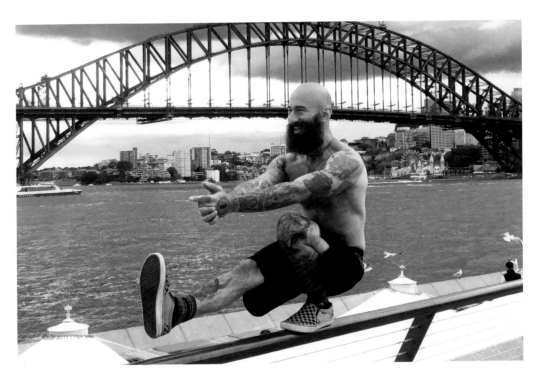

I'm advancing faster with certain exercises than others. Is it okay to mix and match different parts of the different phases of the program?

Absolutely. We wanted to give our readers as detailed of a program as possible, but there's no one-size-fits-all template that will cause everyone who follows it to progress in exactly the same fashion. Some may find that they are ready to move on to more advanced lower-body exercises but are still working with beginner pull-up progressions; others may experience the opposite. Just be careful that you don't fall into the habit of only training your strengths while ignoring your weaknesses. It might be more fun to train the exercises that you are better at, but it's also important to aim for a well-rounded physique.

I've been stuck on the same phase of the program for a long time. No matter how hard I train, I feel like I'm not getting anywhere. What can I do to bust through this plateau?

We all progress at different rates, but everyone who works out consistently for long enough will at some point hit a plateau. It can be frustrating when your training does not advance as seamlessly as you would like it to, but progress is never a straight line.

Also remember that there are ways to gauge your development other than adding reps. If you've been training consistently, it is likely that your body awareness and exercise technique are improving. Pay attention to see if you feel more in control of your movements. Try not to get too hung up on the numbers.

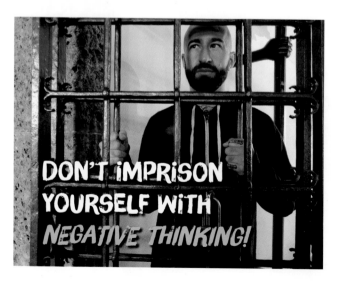

Your mental attitude will also play an important role in your progress. Positive thinking can do wonders for your workouts. Stop telling yourself that you are on a plateau and start believing that you are going to get strong. Don't imprison yourself with negative thinking!

Why is Danny bigger than you? He must be hitting the weights, right?

Danny has more mass than I do, but lifting weights has nothing to do with it. Though we share the same parents and the same gene pool, we are not identical twins and did not get the exact same genetic make-up. Danny's shoulders are broader than mine, his hips are wider and his wrists are thicker. He's also an inch taller and outweighs me by about 20 pounds. Plus he's got a full head of hair. Our bodies do not look exactly alike, even though we're brothers who share very similar lifestyles and training practices. It's hard for some people to accept it, but even though Danny and I have a lot in common, we're also different.

But who's stronger?

Strength is not always so cut and dry. Danny is stronger at certain things. I am stronger at others. Life is full of contradictions. Just because something is true, that doesn't mean the opposite can't also be true. Things are not always black and white.

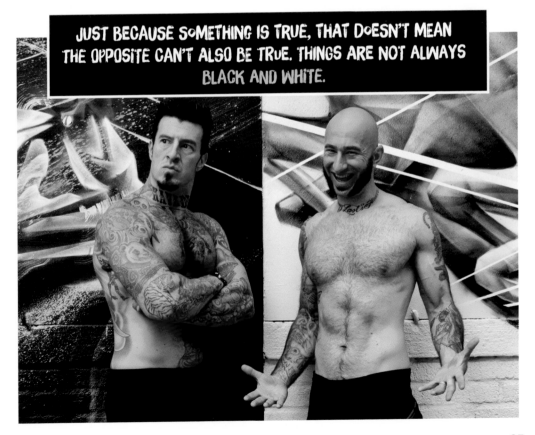

> JUST BECAUSE SOMETHING IS TRUE, THAT DOESN'T MEAN THE OPPOSITE CAN'T ALSO BE TRUE. THINGS ARE NOT ALWAYS BLACK AND WHITE.

Should I do something at the end of my workout to cool down?

Not necessarily, though you can repeat any or all of the warm-up exercises at the end of your training, too. You may also include additional stretches if you like.

I read that it's best to go very slowly during your exercises when practicing calisthenics for strength. Is this true?

My take on rep tempo is that you should aim to be in control of every aspect of your movements, regardless of speed. Oftentimes, when we rush through our reps, the quality declines. For this reason, I urge you to take your time when performing these exercises. However, as your strength and control increases, you may be able to complete your reps a bit quicker without sacrificing your form. Though a pistol squat will obviously take longer than a push-up, when you've truly conquered an exercise, you should be able to do it at just about any tempo with precision and control.

You guys have some awesome ink! I want to get a tattoo but I'm worried it will get warped after I gain some muscle. Should I wait until after I've added a few inches to my arms?

When your arms grow, it's the skin around the armpit that shows the evidence. Take a look at the location of stretch marks on people who have had rapid changes in their weight. They're almost always near the armpits. So if you get a tattoo on your arm, even with substantial muscular growth, there is only so much your tattoo can realistically enlarge. I got my first tattoo on my shoulder when I was just 15 years old. I've added a couple of inches to my arms since then, but the tattoo has held up pretty well, especially considering it's now older than a lot of my readers!

*I'm following the **Get Strong** program and even doing some additional push-ups, but my chest is not developing as much as I'd like. I want my chest to look like yours, Al! Got any tips?*

Push-ups are my number one exercise for the chest, but it's important to remember that individual genetics play a major factor in the shape of your muscles. Some people's chests tend to develop differently than others, regardless of how they train. It's important to learn to love your body for what it is, instead of harping on perceived imperfections. Your chest might not ever look exactly like mine and that's okay. But if you keep training hard, you will become a stronger, buffer version of *you*. Be cool and focus on your training. In time, the aesthetics will fall into place.

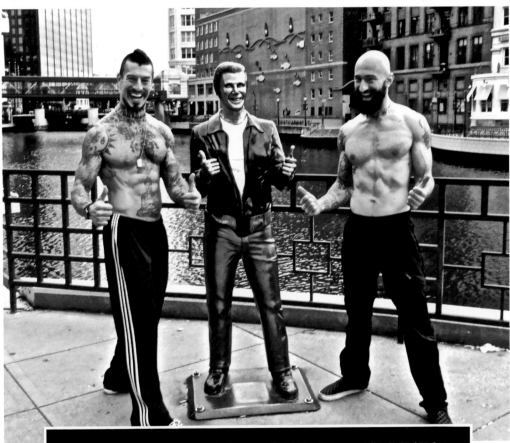

BE *COOL* AND FOCUS ON YOUR TRAINING.

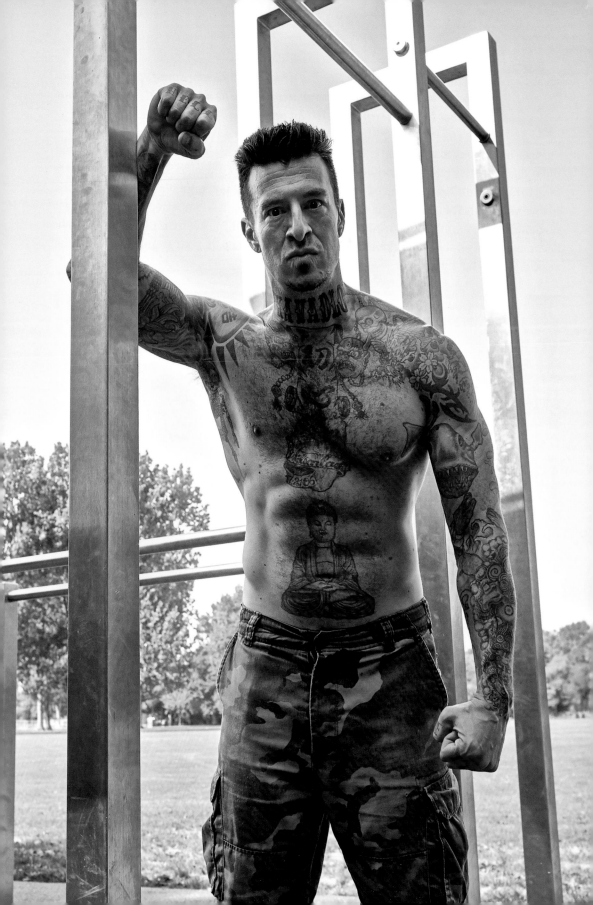

DANNY'S DOS AND DON'TS

 ## DO SEE IT THROUGH

The path to physical fitness is a venture upon which many citizens of the world aspire to embark. Out of this group, very few actually get started. Of those who do find the gumption to begin, even fewer continue. Such is human nature.

Much of the time, actions seem accessible when they exist solely as hypothetical desires, but they become far more difficult when the time comes to put them into practice. What many individuals fail to understand is that exercise is very much a continued practice.

Within said practice, there will frequently and consistently be moments of self-doubt, laziness or perceived impossibility. You may even experience feelings of desperation or despair. I'd be lying if I told you that I've never thought of throwing in the proverbial towel. Even the greatest of champions have moments where they feel they cannot go on. But I encourage you to go on anyway.

The **Get Strong** program is designed to take you from the very beginning of your strength training journey and leave you forged from steel. But you have to see it through. Nothing great can be accomplished without discipline and dedication. Hard work, consistency and patience are the ingredients for success. So when you have those moments of weakness, as we all occasionally do, you must rise above. The program works, but only if you do it. In fact, this sentiment applies to life and every single endeavor we begin. If we do not see things through in our training, careers, aspirations or romantic desires, then we are selling ourselves dangerously and irresponsibly short.

DO ADOPT HEALTHY
DAY-TO-DAY HABITS

In the 1976 motion picture *Taxi Driver,* Travis Bickle as portrayed by Robert De Niro states: "You're only as healthy as you feel" before he begins training to get in the finest shape of his life. Yes, Mr. Bickle does make some questionable judgments in the film, such as trying to assassinate a politician, befriending an underage prostitute and bringing a young lady to a porn theatre for their first date, but the decision to get fit is NOT one of them. In order for us to feel healthy (and be healthy), we must adopt healthy habits.

Just doing the workouts is not always enough. If we're training three to four hours a week, there is still a great deal of time when poor decision making can send us into a downward spiral. In other words, we are the product of the practices we do on a daily basis, so it's important to take care of yourself even when you're not training.

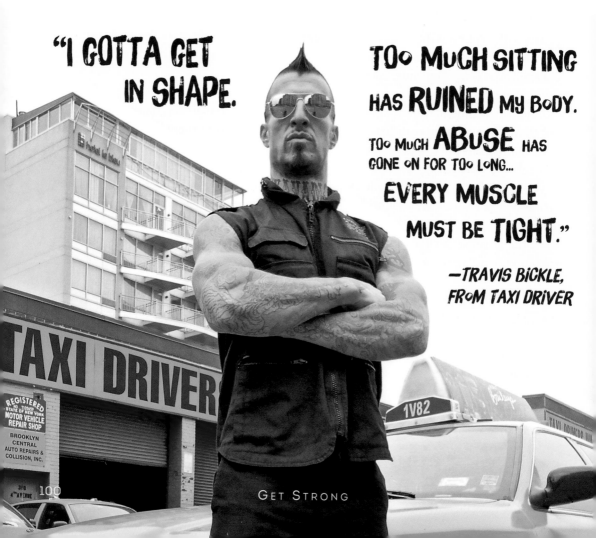

"I GOTTA GET
IN SHAPE.

TOO MUCH SITTING
HAS RUINED MY BODY.
TOO MUCH ABUSE HAS
GONE ON FOR TOO LONG...
EVERY MUSCLE
MUST BE TIGHT."

—TRAVIS BICKLE,
FROM TAXI DRIVER

GET STRONG

Yes, taking the time to perform push-ups, pull-ups and squats is fantastic! But one cannot be sedentary, destructive and completely unaccountable the rest of the time, and expect a dramatically positive outcome.

That's right; even if you train frequently and intensely, if you do not treat yourself well the rest of the time, there is only so much those few hours a week can do to rectify it. If you're eating low quality food often, being inactive most of the time, not getting enough sleep or consuming too many toxins, then expect consequences and understand the reasons why. It is not that the training isn't working, but simply that it cannot offset too many hours of self-abuse.

I cannot tell you how many times I have come across well meaning individuals who experience back pain, for example, and blame it on the one hour that they worked out, without ever considering the sixty hours that they spent seated on their posterior, slouching over a desk. It's backwards logic. Exercise makes you stronger and more vital, not weaker and in greater pain.

 # DO WORK ON IMPROVING YOUR TECHNIQUE

"How do you get to Carnagie Hall?", beckons the old joke.

The answer, of course, is "Practice."

Well, exercise takes practice, too. I am often asked, "What's the next progression after you can do a human flag?" Here's the answer: "Do a better human flag."

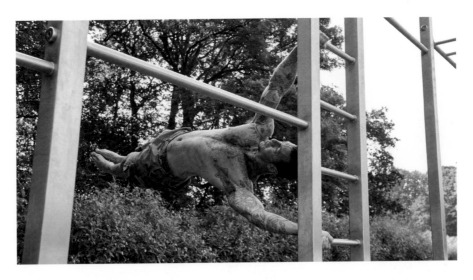

You see, while it's true that you never forget your first time, nobody's first is their best. (This applies to events other than exercise as well.) We strive to get better over time. Your first archer pull-up, push-up or one leg squat may indeed be in need of improvement. After you do that first one, then work on doing it better. I refer to this as "technical progression" which is, in and of itself, a form of increasing the difficulty of any exercise. The first step to doing something well is often just to get it done, but ultimately, we want to be greater than that.

 ## DO SPREAD THE WORD

When the *Get Strong* program works for you, it is not only your right to let others know, it is also your responsibility. Spreading the word is part of why I got started in the fitness industry in the first place. I had personally helped a great number of people who professed to me how happy they were to finally take their health seriously. Much of the time their only regret was that they wished they'd started sooner. I still encounter people every day who express this to me.

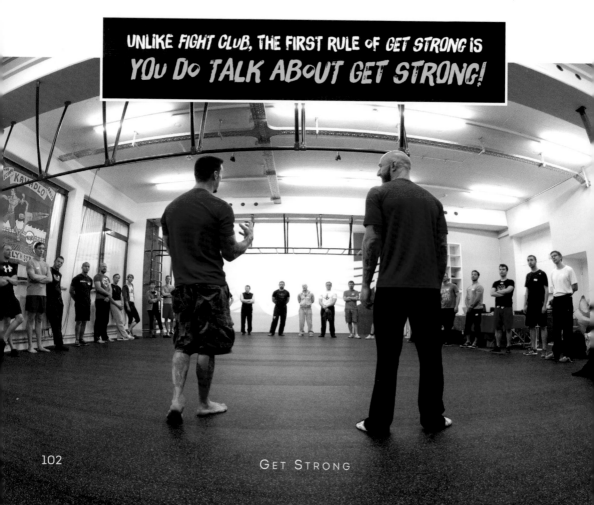

UNLIKE *FIGHT CLUB*, THE FIRST RULE OF *GET STRONG* IS YOU DO TALK ABOUT GET STRONG!

Think about how much better you feel when you're active and healthy than when you're not. Shouldn't everyone feel this good? Well, they can. It's up to you to help.

One of the greatest aspects of the calisthenics community is the support, encouragement and nurturing that we give to each other. Sometimes, sadly, newcomers are under the mistaken impression that the fitness world is some private club, but the truth is that everybody is welcome here. We want to celebrate each individual's success, regardless of his or her current fitness level. That's why the *Get Strong* program starts from the very beginning. It's geared toward the novice as well as the advanced practitioner.

If you know anyone who can benefit from this book, then tell them about it. Carry it with you. Share it with your friends. Post about it online. Unlike *Fight Club*, the first rule of *Get Strong* is you DO talk about *Get Strong*!

DO LEARN FROM YOUR MISTAKES

Even when doing the best we can, we must acknowledge that nobody is immune to gaffe. Yes, the greatest heroes, protectors and role models have been known at times to fall from grace. It's okay; I forgive them. I myself, am so far from perfect, it's ridiculous. Don't put me or anyone else on a pedestal. We are all human.

Like I tell my son when he makes a mistake: "Add up how many times you've messed up and then multiply it by a thousand. That's how many times I've messed up."

There is nothing wrong with messing up. It's how we learn.

Sometimes losses, failures and transgressive behaviors are merely the cost of doing business. The virtue lies in learning from these errors and coming back better and stronger from it. Oftentimes the wisdom and experience we earn from our misjudgments surpasses the savvy we attribute to our successes.

X DON'T BE AFRAID TO MAKE CHANGES WHEN NEEDED

Even if you fall off, don't quit. Get back in it. This notion remains true for the *Get Strong* program as well as for life. Sometimes adjustments are needed.

If circumstances prohibit you from doing the prescribed number of workouts, if you skip a day, or even a week, then pick yourself up, dust yourself off and get back on the program.

As much as we have the desire to rule our own universe, there will always be factors for which we simply did not plan. You may be caught up in family responsibilities, work obligations, legal issues or other commitments. Still, there are ways to find the time.

If this is the case, then I, Danny Kavadlo, am personally giving you permission to adjust the program if it's necessary to fit it into your life. This is how we create time for things that are important to us: by improvising when we have to. To put it in practical, actionable terms, if you need to repeat Phase 3, Week 2 before moving onto Week 3, then do it!

As long as you're doing the work, you will get results. The important sentiment is to keep a positive mental attitude and maintain a continued commitment. Stay on track and tough it out, which brings me to my next point...

X DON'T GO AWAY MAD

Finish every set on a good rep. Don't conclude your workout with something you feel you could have done better. End on a high note.

This is another assertion that can be applied not only to our workouts, but also to other areas of life. Don't go to bed angry at your partner. Tell them you love them and kiss them goodnight. Don't quit your job in an epic screaming match with your boss. Give proper notice and do your work to the best of your ability until it is time for your departure. Don't hang up on your friend just because you are having an argument at that time. Acknowledge that the conversation is going nowhere and peacefully get off the phone. Negativity will eat you up from the inside out every single time, so foster positive energy in the best way you can. You'll be glad you did. No one has ever regretted taking the high road.

X DON'T ENTRUST YOUR FORTUNE TO YOUR MEMORY

I remember it well. It was Friday, June 7, 2013. It was the world's first ever Progressive Calisthenics Certification. We stood in a large recreation center, a gymnasium of sorts, deep in the inner-city of Minneapolis, Minnesota.

The room was packed. The air stood still. Emotions ran high. Something legendary was about to go down. And that was the first time I heard it...

My publisher, mentor and (I'm proud to say) dear friend Mr. John Du Cane, CEO of Dragon Door Publications, facilitator of greatness and modern-day fitness revolutionary, spoke these seven true words:

"Don't entrust your fortune to your memory."

Mr. Du Cane was referring to the importance of writing things down. You see, when you attend a Progressive Calisthenics Certification, you are not only bombarded with community, passion and spirit, you are also given a boatload of expert information. It's a lot to absorb!

As human beings, we have limitations. Our memory is often one of them. How many times have you been walking down the street and you are struck with a great notion? You swear you will remember it because it's so true, so honest and so important. But you don't.

You should have written it down. Mr. Du Cane was right.

I am proud to say that I've heard John Du Cane say these words scores more times at PCC certifications all over the world and it never gets old. In fact, I am always grateful to hear it.

And now I'm finally writing it down.

✗ DON'T GIVE UP

Hellyeah it hurts. Sometimes all we know is pain, but it is only through our pain that we can ultimately summon prosperity. No matter how hard you get hit, you need to move forward. To channel Byron, "The heart will break, but broken live on."

The decision to cease or proceed is yours and only yours to make. At the end of the day, when you lie in your bed naked, cold and exposed, you alone decide whether to stop or continue. Nobody gets a vote but you.

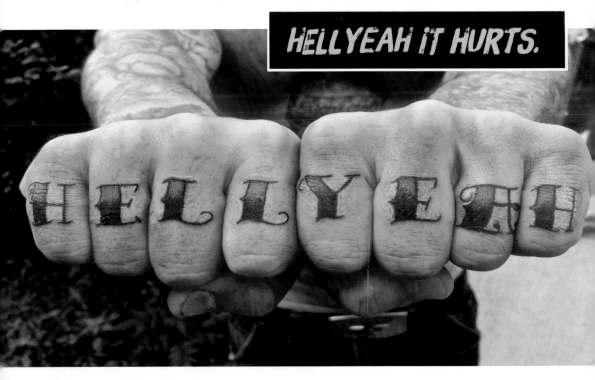

✗ DON'T LET THE HATERS BRING YOU DOWN

There will always be haters in all walks of life. In the fitness world, it used to be limited to some know-it-all in the gym loudly declaring, "You're doing it wrong!" In the Internet age, unconstructive criticism is more rampant than ever. Many times, folks will hide behind their keyboards and offer everything from misinformed advice to plain old cruelty. All I can say is, don't take the bait. Adversity breeds adversity and it's the bearers of such malevolence that pay the price, so don't play into it.

After all, it takes two. Everything does. The haters dish it out, but their antagonism won't have a leg to stand on if you choose not to receive it. Don't give life to their fruitless hostility. If you pay them no mind, then their comments will cease to exist in your world. No one can dance with an unwilling partner.

In the realm of fitness, *all* goals are good goals, and we all do better when we support one another. There's too much to love in this world to get sucked into the hate. So get out there and train hard. It's time to **Get Strong**!

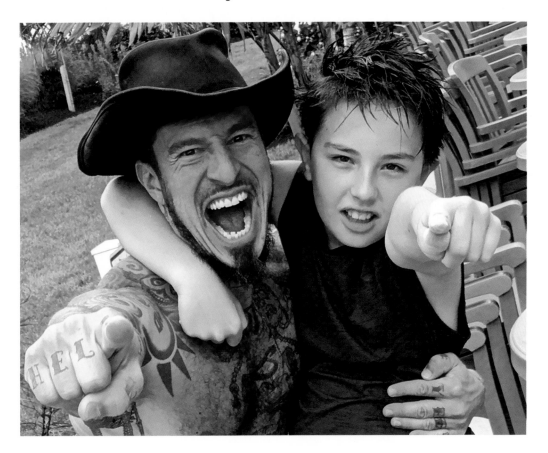

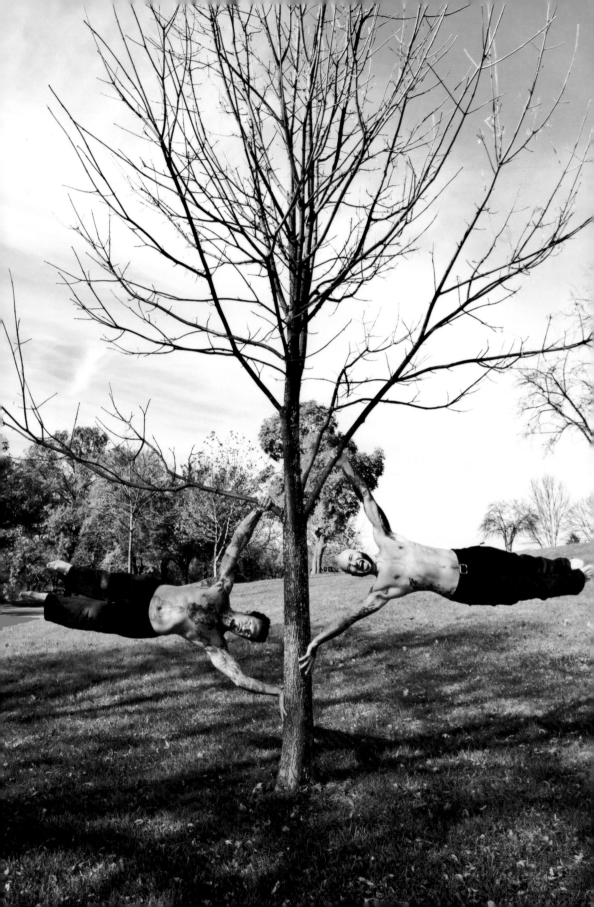

SUPPLEMENTAL EXERCISES

There is an endless universe of calisthenics exercises in existence. The ones that follow are not included in the **Get Strong** program because, honestly, you can get strong without them. That said, there is always a virtue in switching things up. We enjoy giving you a broad palette from which to paint and these are some of the best moves around that truly represent strength.

Some of these exercises call for more equipment (such as a vertical pole or a set of parallel bars) than those included in the **Get Strong** program. You will find some of them to be basic and fundamental, while others will be more exotic and advanced. Aussie pull-ups and dips, for example, are foundational strength exercises, while the human flag and front lever are elite level feats of strength. All of these moves are worth exploring in your pursuit of bodyweight mastery.

AUSSIE PULL-UP

1   Get down under a bar that's about waist height with your legs extended in front of you to form a straight line from the back of your head to your heels.

2   Grip the bar firmly and brace your entire body as you pull your chest toward the bar. Be careful not to bend your hips or shrug your shoulders.

3   Pause briefly at the top, with your chest approximately 1-2 inches from the bar, then lower yourself back to the bottom with control.

Trainer Talk: If you are unable to perform this exercise on a bar of waist height, it may be helpful to use a higher bar.

Muscles Emphasized: Lats, biceps.

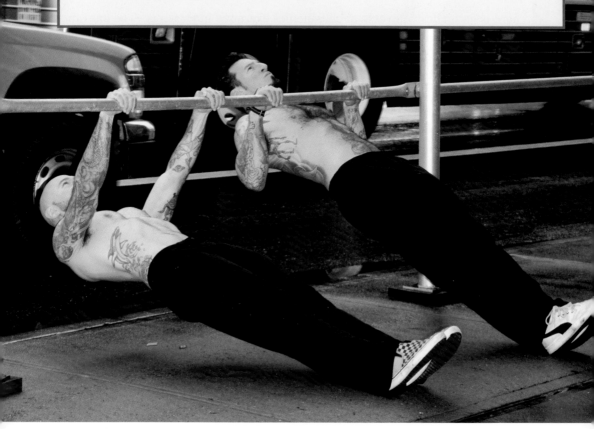

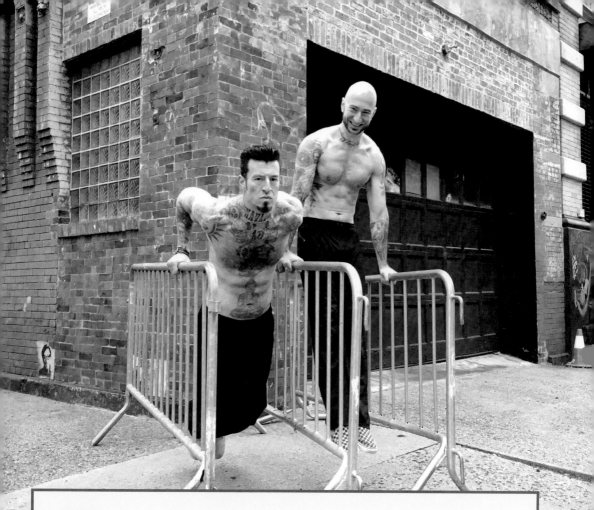

DIP

1   Position yourself upright between two parallel bars with your feet off the floor.

2   Brace your trunk and bend from your shoulders and elbows, lowering yourself until your elbows are bent to at least 90 degrees.

3   Pause briefly at the bottom, then press yourself back to the top.

Trainer Talk: *Make sure your elbows point behind you instead of flaring out to the sides. This will keep tension on your triceps and minimize shearing forces on your shoulders.*

Muscles Emphasized: *Triceps, shoulders, chest.*

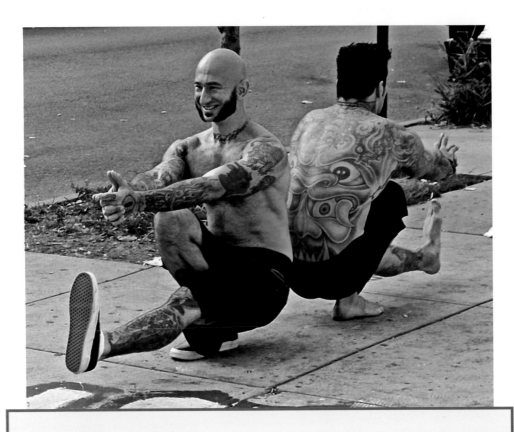

PISTOL SQUAT

1   Stand upright and lift one leg in the air with your knee fully
    extended.

2   Reach your arms forward and bend from the hip, knee and an-
    kle of your standing leg to squat down as low as possible.

3   Pause when your hamstrings come in contact with your calf,
    keeping tension in your abs, then return to the top position.
    Complete your set in its entirety and then repeat on the
    other leg.

Trainer Talk: Don't be surprised if you feel your non-squatting leg
          working during a pistol squat. You will need to engage
          your hip flexors and quadriceps on that side in order to
          keep your leg extended in the air.

Muscles Emphasized: Quadriceps, hamstrings, glutes, abs.

MUSCLE-UP

1 Hang from an overhead bar with an overhand grip, positioning your hands slightly narrower than you would for a pull-up.

2 Lean back and pull the bar all the way down to your sternum. At the top of your pull, reach your chest over the bar and extend your arms.

3 Pause here briefly before lowering back down to the bottom position.

Trainer Talk:
It can take some practice to get a feel for the timing of this exercise, so be patient. When starting out, we encourage you to use momentum and be explosive in order to get your torso above the bar. Over time, you'll learn to rely less on momentum to get to the top position.

Muscles Emphasized:
Lats, shoulders, chest, biceps, triceps, abs.

L-SIT

1   Sit on the floor with your palms on the ground and your legs
    fully extended in front of you.

2   Press your hands into the ground and raise your bottom and
    legs off the floor. Make sure to keep your legs locked out at the
    knees and fully extended.

3   Hold this pose for time and return to the seated position.

Trainer Talk: It can be helpful for beginners to perform this exercise
on an elevated surface. As the L-sit requires a high de-
gree of flexibility in the hamstrings, the elevation will
allow you to let your legs drop slightly below hip level
if needed.

Muscles Emphasized: Abs, hip flexors, shoulders, triceps,
quadriceps, wrists.

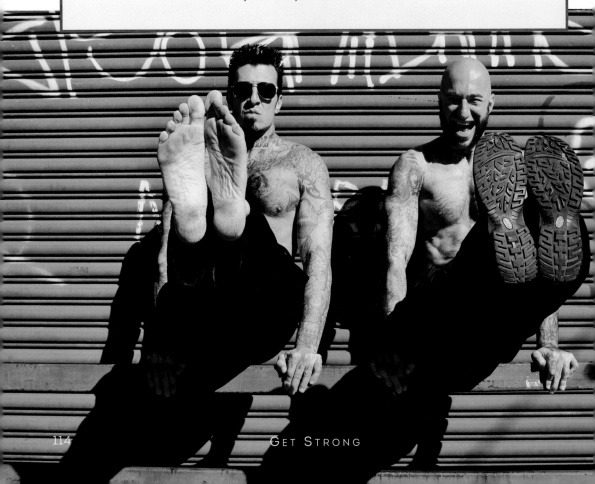

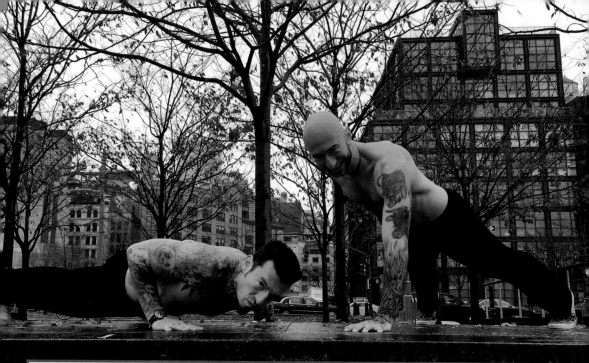

ONE ARM PUSH-UP

1   *Start in a push-up position, only with your feet farther apart and your hands closer together. Keep tension throughout your entire body and remove one hand from the floor, placing it at your side.*

2   *Bend your grounded arm and lower your chest toward the floor, making sure to keep your elbow close to your side. Keep your shoulders even, without bending or waiving at the hips.*

3   *Pause briefly with your chest approximately one inch from the ground, then press yourself back to the top, maintaining tension in your abs, glutes and legs the entire time. Complete your set in its entirety and then repeat on the other side.*

Trainer Talk: *Beginners will find this exercise more accessible if they perform it with their hand on an elevated surface. The change in leverage will place less weight in the hand. The higher the surface, the more mechanically forgiving the exercise becomes.*

Muscles Emphasized: *Chest, shoulders, triceps, abs.*

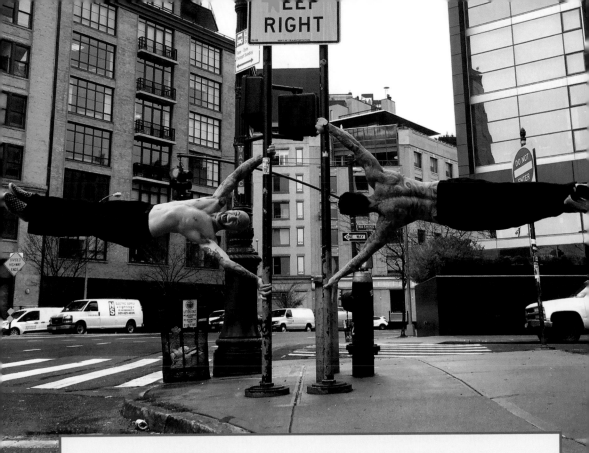

HUMAN FLAG

1   Place your hands slightly wider than shoulder width apart on a vertical pole or other stable vertical object.

2   Keeping your bottom arm locked and your grip tight, kick up into a horizontal position with your body perpendicular to the pole. Brace every muscle in your body as you press with your bottom arm and pull with your top arm.

3   Hold this position and repeat on the other side.

Trainer Talk: Keeping your body at a slightly lower (or higher) angle and/or tucking one or both knees are good ways to train until you are capable of achieving the full human flag.

Muscles Emphasized: Lats, shoulders, biceps, triceps, grip, abs, glutes.

FRONT LEVER

1   Begin in the active hang position.

2   Keep your elbows locked and squeeze the bar tightly as you pull your body up until it is parallel to the ground. It can be helpful to envision driving the bar down toward your hips. Flex your lats, abs, glutes and quadriceps in order to maintain a straight body.

3   Hold this position, then lower yourself back down.

Trainer Talk: Keeping your body at a slightly lower (or higher) angle and/or tucking one or both knees are good ways to train until you are capable of achieving the full front lever.

Muscles Emphasized: Lats, shoulders, biceps, triceps, grip, abs, glutes.

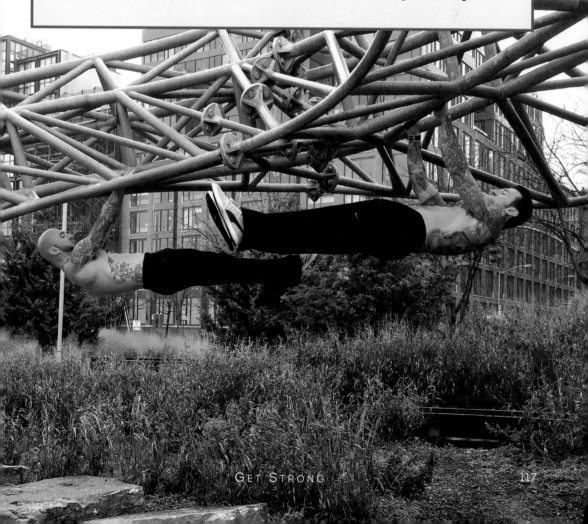

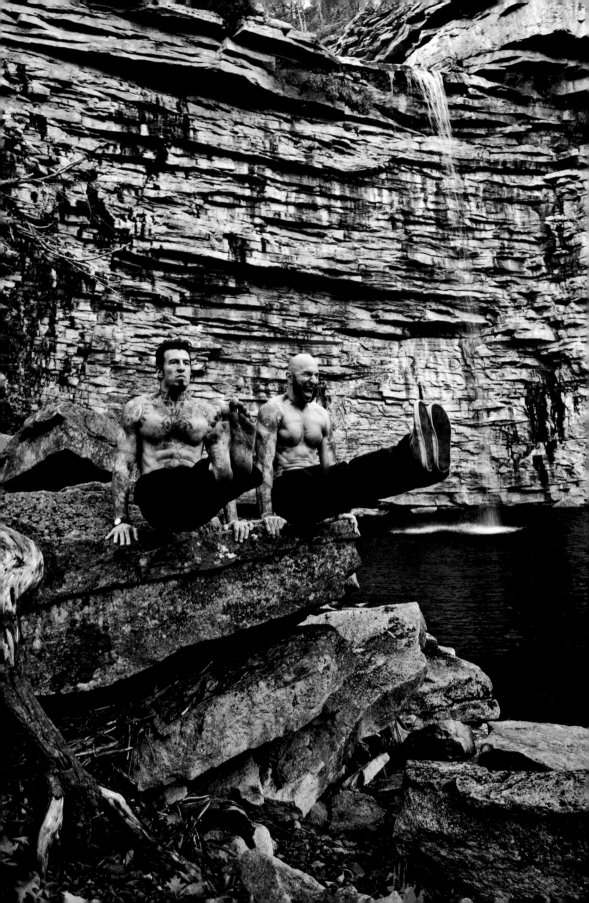

SUPPLEMENTAL WORKOUTS

The workouts in the *Get Strong* program provide all you need. If your goal is to be strong, ripped and powerful, you already have the tools. The program works.

For the sake of variety, however, you may want to try some different routines over the course of time. The desire and ability to adapt and change is an important part of life. As you know by now, when we train using a minimalist methodology, we open ourselves up to endless possibilities.

Feel free to follow these workouts as written, or modify them to suit your preferences.

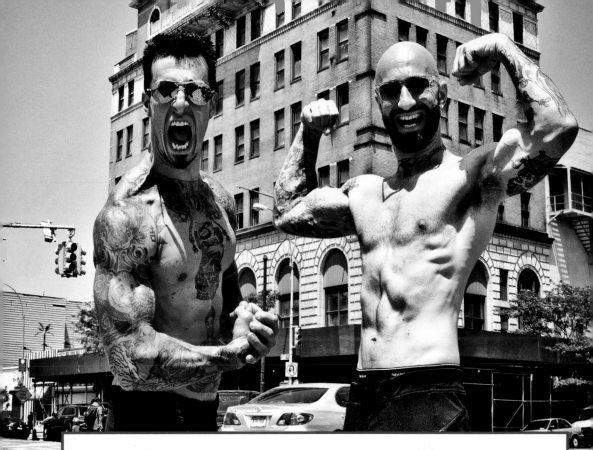

Suns Out, Guns Out

This intermediate level upper-body workout will give your arms a nice pump and build real-world strength that's sure to carry over into all sorts of summer-time fun!

When you perform exercises that employ compound movements, you can target multiple muscle groups at once. In addition to your arms, this workout will hit your entire upper body, even your abs.

Push-up	3 x 20 reps
Dip	3 x 20 reps
Chin-up	3 x 10 reps
Aussie Pull-up	3 x 10 reps
Feet Elevated Pike Push-up	3 x 10 reps
Wall Handstand	3 x 30 seconds

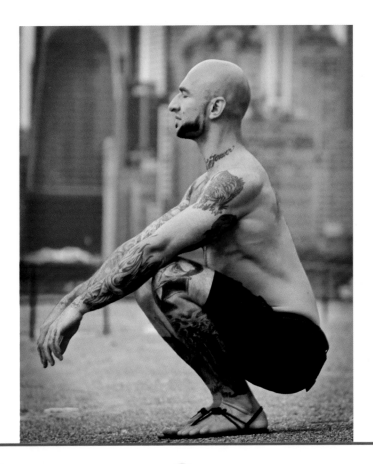

WHEELS OF STEEL

This intermediate level lower-body workout will rev your engine and get your wheels turning. As your legs contain the largest muscles in your body, they require lots of oxygen and blood flow. Therefore, this workout will challenge your heart and lungs in addition to every muscle in your lower body. Remember, if you don't have strong legs, you're not strong.

Squat	2 x 20 reps
Step-up	2 x 20 reps (10 per leg)
Bulgarian Split Squat	2 x 20 reps (10 per leg)
Drinking Bird	2 x 20 reps (10 per leg)
Candlestick Bridge	2 x 20 reps (10 per leg)

ABSOLUTE ZERO

This is the perfect beginner/intermediate level workout for when you find yourself with absolutely no equipment to use for your training. These five classic calisthenics exercises will always be available to you, regardless of the circumstances.

You can still get a great full body workout with nothing but the ground beneath your feet.

Squat	2 x 20 reps
Push-up	2 x 20 reps
Hip Bridge	2 x 20 reps
Split Squat	2 x 20 reps (10 per leg)
Lying Knee Tuck	2 x 20 reps

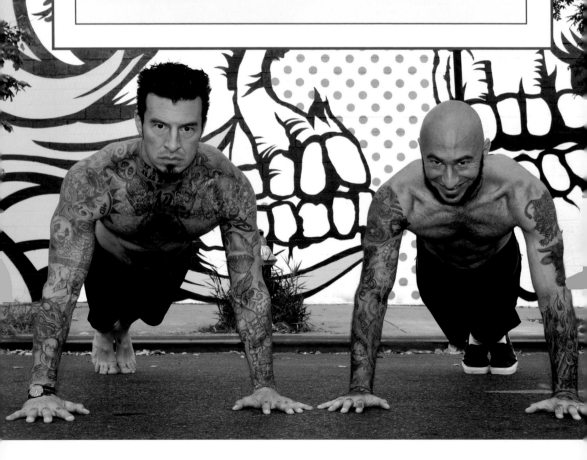

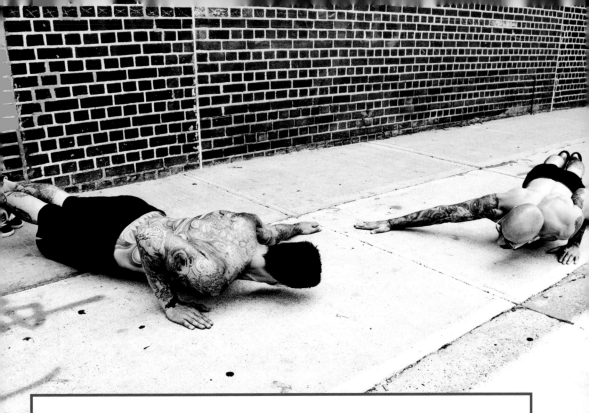

ZERO TOLERANCE

Here is an intermediate/advanced level workout that requires zero equipment. Even after your tolerance for exercise has increased, you can still train your entire body using only the floor. Never judge the difficulty of a workout by how much equipment it calls for.

Archer Squat	2 x 20 reps (10 per leg)
Archer Push-up	2 x 20 reps (10 per arm)
Candlestick Straight Bridge	2 x 20 reps (10 per leg)
Hover Lunge	2 x 20 reps (10 per leg)
Drinking Bird	2 x 20 reps (10 per leg)
L-sit	2 x 20 seconds

PISTOL PREP

This workout will help you build the strength and control to perform a full pistol squat. The first two exercises warm up your legs and prepare you for the single leg movements that follow.

When performing the assisted one leg squats, use the lowest elevated surface that you can without significantly sacrificing your form. Aim to gradually reduce the height of the surface. When performing the one leg squats, keep your non-squatting leg as close to parallel to the ground as possible. These methods will help you get closer to the full pistol squat.

If you cannot perform each exercise in a single set, then break them up as needed. As long as you get all the work done, you are on the right track.

Squat	2 x 20 reps
Archer Squat	2 x 20 reps (10 per leg)
Assisted One Leg Squat	2 x 20 reps (10 per leg)
One Leg Squat	3 x 10 reps (5 per leg)

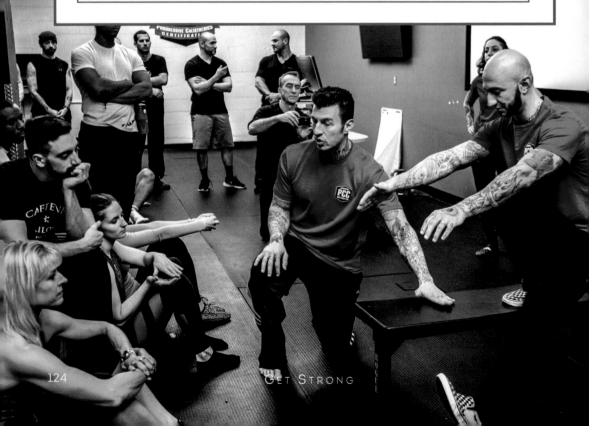

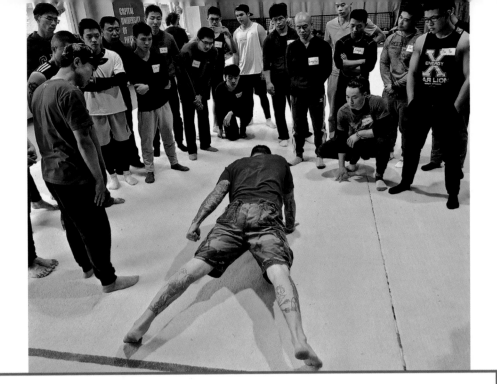

O.A.P. Academy

This workout will help you build the strength and control to perform a full one arm push-up. The first two exercises warm up your arms and prepare you for the single arm movements that follow.

When performing the archer push-ups, use your primary arm as much as possible. With practice, you'll work toward gradually reducing the amount of assistance needed from the opposite arm. When performing the hand elevated one arm push-ups, use the lowest elevated surface that you can, without significantly sacrificing your form. Aim to gradually reduce the height of the surface. These methods will help you get closer to the full one arm push-up.

If you cannot perform each exercise in a single set, feel free to break them up as needed. As long as you get all the work done, you are on the right track.

Push-up	2 x 20 reps
Archer Push-up	2 x 10 reps (5 per arm)
Hand Elevated One Arm Push-up	3 x 10 reps (5 per arm)

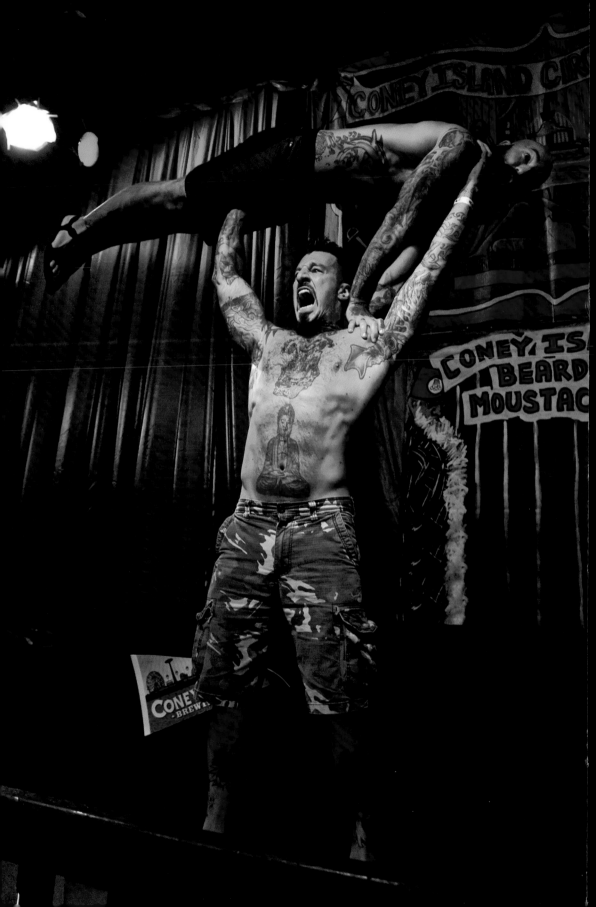

PARTNER EXERCISES

We always encourage our bodyweight buddies to spread the word about calisthenics, but getting your friends to join you is even better. If you have a partner and need a break from your usual routine, you can mix things up by practicing partner exercises that use one another's bodies as training equipment.

Though the exercises discussed in Part I can be enough to keep you busy for a lifetime, the realm of partner bodyweight training opens up an entirely new avenue to explore. Admittedly, some of these moves have more of a novelty element to them than others, but there is still a lot of practical value here. When performing coordinated bodyweight exercises in tandem with another human being, the proprioceptive challenges are increased, and you are forced to pay closer attention not only to your own movements, but to those of your partner as well.

The following exercises are all about communication and working as a team. Both parties must use their entire bodies in distinct ways to achieve success in this arena. Anytime you're learning to move your body in new ways it's great for your mind as well as your muscles.

Remember to switch roles with your partner when practicing these exercises, as each person's role is different within each move, and experiencing both sides of the equation will lead to a better training session.

Though the degree of difficulty varies significantly between the following exercises, once you have established a baseline of strength and body awareness, you can have fun playing with these partner variants. So grab a friend and let's get started.

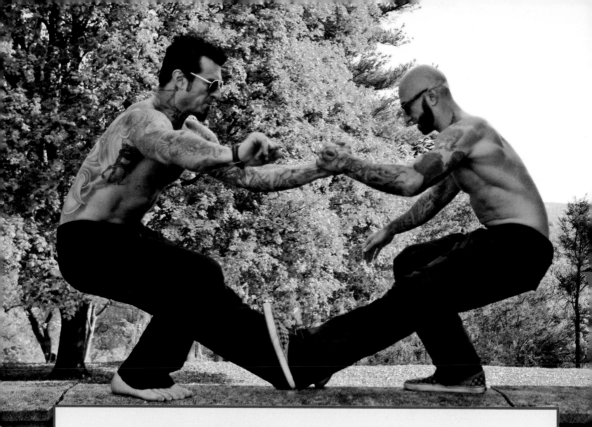

PARTNER PISTOL

Face your partner and clasp hands while you both lift one leg in the air and extend it in front of your body. Make sure you both lift the same leg so you don't kick each other. (If your partner lifts his or her right leg, then you lift your right leg as well.) You may also need to stagger your stance a bit to avoid getting in the way of one another.

From this position, both of you will lower down into the deepest single-leg squat you can manage, using your partner to maintain stability and balance. Make sure to go slowly and avoid using momentum to drop down. Pause briefly at the bottom, then squeeze your partner's hand, clench your abs and drive the heel of your squatting leg into the floor to stand up. When you finish one side, switch and repeat on the other leg.

In this modification of the pistol squat, you and your partner provide increased stability for each other as well as a counterbalance, making this difficult move a more manageable task for you both. The partner pistol can be a very useful step toward achieving a full, unassisted pistol squat.

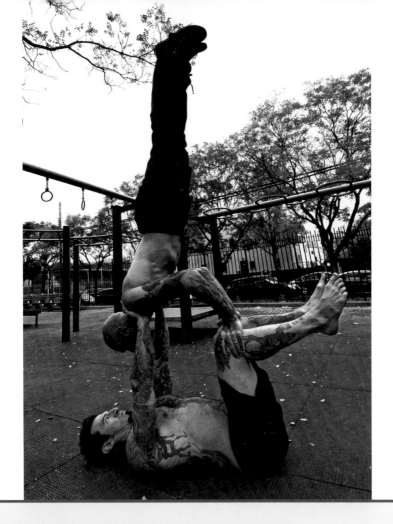

PARTNER SHOULDER STAND

Begin on your back, with both arms extended in the air above your chest. Lift your feet with your knees bent to around 90 degrees, then have your partner stand below you and grab the tops of your shins. From there, they will lower their upper traps/shoulders into your hands and begin shifting their weight forward off of their feet. Keeping your elbows locked, press away from your chest like you are locking out a push-up as your partner shifts their weight entirely into your hands. The person on top should aim to get their hips in the air above their shoulders, eventually lifting themselves into a full inversion, supported only on the knees and hands of their partner.

This bodyweight inversion is a fun way to get a challenging workout as well as build trust and camaraderie.

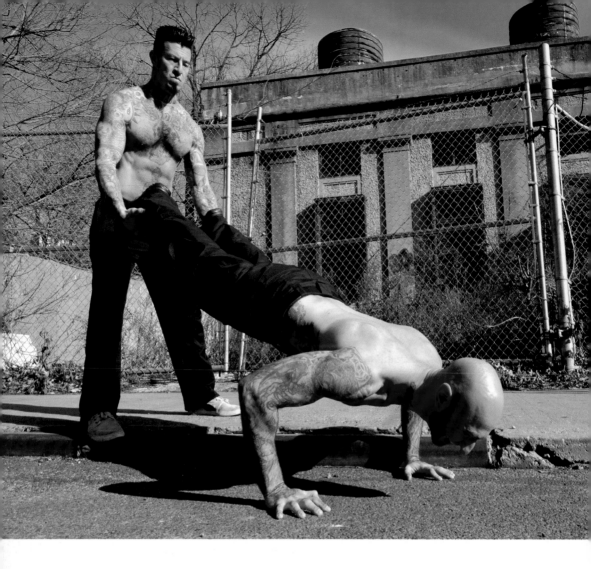

WHEELBARROW PUSH-UP

Begin in the top of a push-up position with your partner holding your ankles. Keeping your hands below your shoulders, carefully lower your chest toward the ground and press yourself back up.

In addition to turning your regular push-up into a feet elevated version, there's a significant amount of instability created by having your partner hold your ankles. The farther from the floor that you get, the less stable the move becomes. Additionally, when your partner holds you up higher, it puts more of your weight in your hands.

HUMAN FLAG AND HUMAN FLAG POLE

Begin by standing to the side of your partner. Grasp their ankle and forearm as they bend their opposite knee, extend their free arm and lean away from you. The arm being grasped should be bent to approximately 90 degrees. Now kick up into a human flag as your partner leans even farther away to counter your weight. It will take some trial and error to find the appropriate balance and tension required.

*This is the exercise that the Kavadlo Brothers first became known for in the calisthenics community. In 2011, we appeared on the cover of Paul "Coach" Wade's **Convict Conditioning 2** performing this feat, which went on to become a signature exercise for us. People all over the world have seen this iconic image immortalized on that legendary cover.*

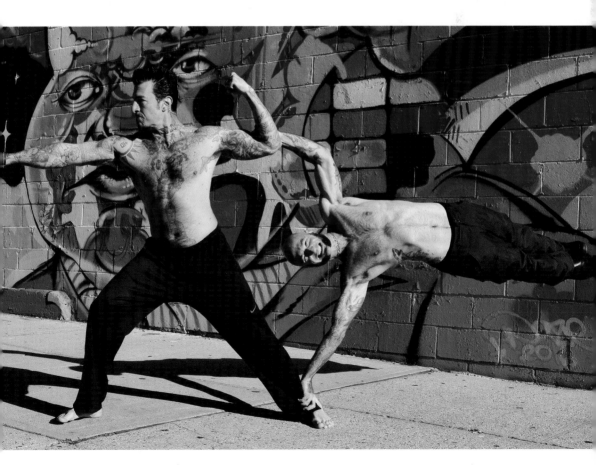

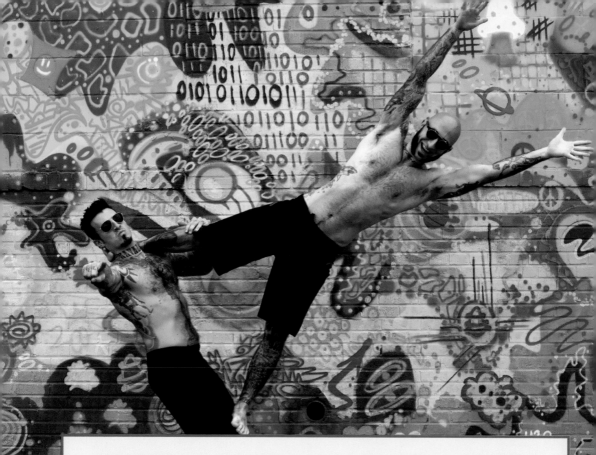

REVERSE HUMAN FLAG & HUMAN FLAG POLE

Begin by having the person who will be the "pole" stand with their feet together and knees partially bent. The flagger will then proceed to hold their partner's hand(s) for stability as they step one foot up on top of their partner's thighs. (Try to keep your feet close to your partner's knees for a more solid foundation.) From there, the flagger will careful-ly slide their opposite foot behind their partner's head. The partner can use his or her hand to help. Now begin extending the body outward, while actively flexing your foot toward the neck of your partner for stability. When both people are ready, you may slowly begin to release your hands.

As with the previous variation, the person acting as the pole must lean in the opposite direction of the flagger in order to provide a coun-terbalance. It is important to lean from the hip and extend from the back, rather than solely at the knees, to provide the right leverage for this balance. Though still a challenging move in its own right, this "foot flag" variant can be more suited to intermediate level practitioners than the previous incarnation, which is very advanced.

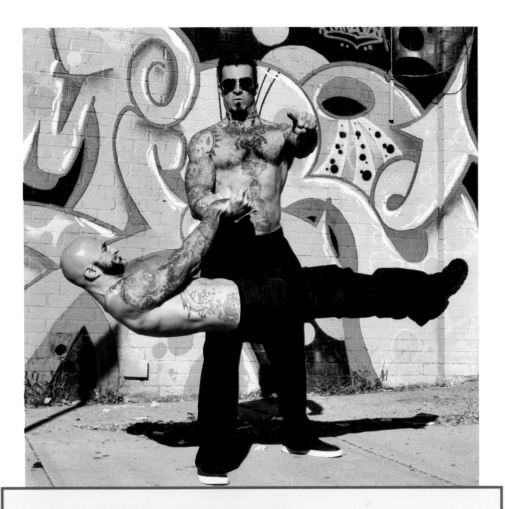

PARTNER FRONT LEVER

Have your partner stand firm, bracing their entire body and bending at the biceps of the arm to be levered upon. Stand in front of them and grip their forearm with all the strength you can muster.

Both partners need to maintain tension in the arms, abs, legs, glutes and shoulders as you enter the front lever position. Keep your arms locked at the elbow and body parallel to the ground.

We've become known for this feat since performing it on the cover of our book **Street Workout**. While the standard front lever is already a difficult bodyweight challenge in its own right, performing it while hanging from another human being can pose an additional challenge.

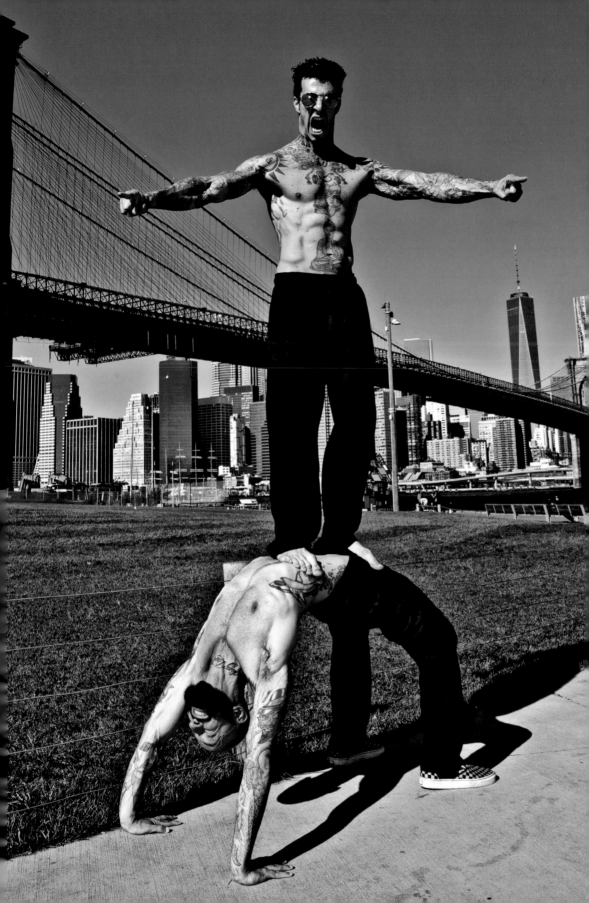

- III -

BONUS
SECTION

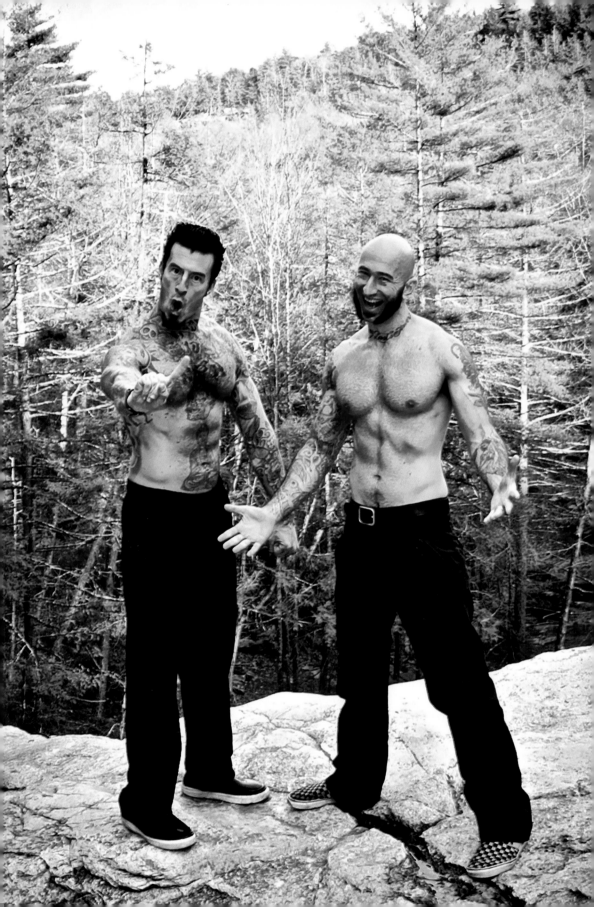

NOW
AND ZEN

*"NO MAN EVER STEPS IN THE SAME RIVER TWICE,
FOR IT'S NOT THE SAME RIVER
AND HE'S NOT THE SAME MAN."*

—HERACLITUS

The Kavadlo Brothers have over 25 years of combined fitness industry experience. Both of us have worn many hats in this business. We've been trainers, authors, models, presenters, consultants and more. We've been in the game for a long time and our passion for fitness has taken us all over the world. In spite of that, we always feel like there's still more to say, still more to do and still more to learn.

Though repetition is part of our job, we've taken a Zen approach to fitness throughout the years, maintaining the "beginner's mind" and the perspective that each experience is happening now for the first time, and the only time. Zen means different things to different people. One way to think of it is living in the moment and fully experiencing reality. Nowadays more than ever, we have a tendency to focus on things that are not in our immediate presence. Whether it's a text message hanging over your head or a load of laundry that needs to be done, we all experience distractions that take us away from what's actually happening around us. Being here now is important.

Zen teaches us to let go of the past, stop worrying about the future and focus on the present. After all, we cannot change the past or predict the future, but by focusing on what's happening now, we are able to take actions that can heal old wounds and allow for our best future to unfold.

But what if—in the present—we take time to reflect. It is often in hindsight that we truly understand the consequences of our actions. Looking back on those effects now can allow us to make more informed decisions.

In the pages ahead, we've revisited some of our past works and given you, our readers and friends, an inside look at our current perspective. We've also added never before seen authors' insights, which provide you with a new context in which to appreciate them, as well as some behind the scenes information on what inspired us to write them in the first place. What follows are ten of our favorite articles that have ever appeared on the web, now in print for the very first time.

This is workout wisdom for the ages. We encourage you to read and reread these articles throughout your fitness journey. You may see something different each time.

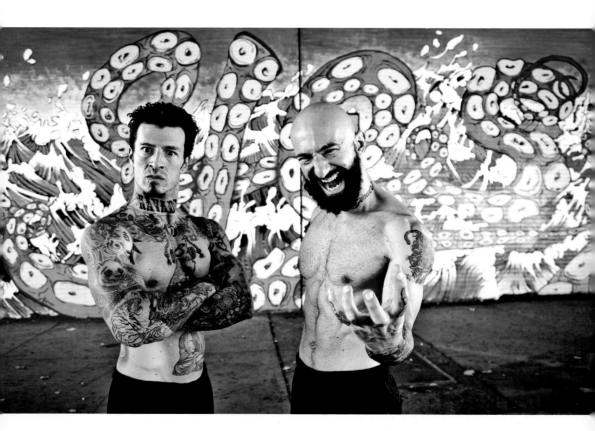

GET STRONG

Actions, Not Words

—By Al Kavadlo

Author's Insight—

I wrote this article soon after the release of my last solo book, *Zen Mind, Strong Body*, as an attempt to further explain the disconnect between theory and practice that has been a key theme in all of my work. More than any particular workout or exercise, the advice in this article is probably the most important lesson I can attempt to impart. The point of these writings is not so much about the words themselves, but rather to inspire you to take action. If I can't get you to do that, then I've failed as a motivator.

> "DON'T THINK, FEEL! IT IS LIKE A FINGER POINTING A WAY
> TO THE MOON. DON'T CONCENTRATE ON THE FINGER
> OR YOU WILL MISS ALL THAT HEAVENLY GLORY."
>
> —BRUCE LEE, FROM *ENTER THE DRAGON*

It may seem obvious, but if you want to get something done, the only way to do so is to take action. You actually have to DO the thing. And it's almost always better to do it sooner rather than later.

Thinking about something is not the same as doing it. Reading about something isn't the same either. Talking certainly isn't doing. In fact, talking is counterproductive in many ways. When you talk about doing something, you scratch your itch to do the thing and you may now be less likely to actually do it. You've alleviated the need to take action in the moment because you just made a plan. (And plans always play out exactly like we want them to, right?) You also feel good because the person you told has probably congratulated you on your decision. Why not celebrate with a cupcake?

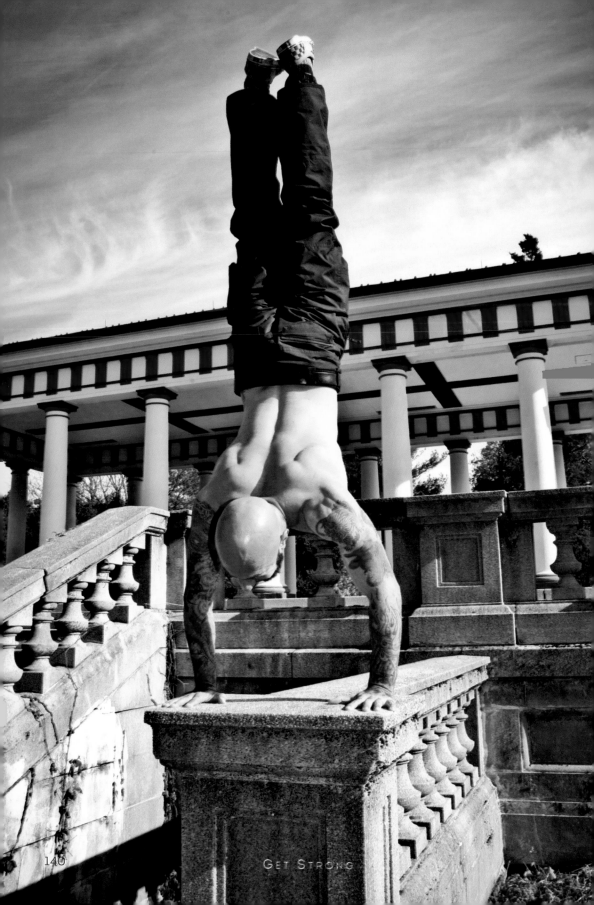

GET STRONG

ZIP IT GOOD

Here's what I want you to try: The next time you decide on a goal for yourself, don't tell ANYONE! Keep it to yourself. If you really feel passionately about this goal, bottling it up will make you think about it more. Thinking about it more will make you more likely to do it. You will want to explode when you finally get the chance to take action. That is, unless you weren't really serious about doing it anyway. If that's the case, it's a good thing you didn't make yourself look foolish by telling all your friends about it and then not following through.

I know, I know. Every book on goal setting tells you to tell your friends about your goals. Telling people gives you accountability, they say. Blah, blah, blah. I already know from over a decade in the personal training industry that that plan doesn't tend to work. Many people talk a good game, but never put their words into action. Talking is talking. Doing is doing. They aren't the same thing.

PSYCH!

Of course there are things in life that we need to mentally psych ourselves up for beforehand. Exercise is usually one of those things. I mentally prepare myself for every one of my workouts. I think about working out, I visualize myself doing it, I project positive thoughts out into the world. I'll even have a template of which exercises I want to do and what order I want to do them in (though I'm also prepared to deviate from that plan if called for). But I don't talk about it—at least not until after I've taken action. When you spend too much time talking about things, you're paralyzed by them. You only learn to walk the path by taking the first step.

One of my favorite Zen parables tells of a great scholar who came to Buddha seeking knowledge. "I have many questions for you," the scholar told Buddha. "I've been told you are the only one who can answer them."

"I will answer all of your questions," replied Buddha. "But before I do that, you must fulfill a requirement. For one year, you must be with me in total silence. I can answer you now, but you are not ready. You must first empty your mind of misconceptions. Study with me in silence for one whole year. Only then will I answer."

The scholar accepted Buddha's offer and began to study under him in silence. After a year had passed, Buddha told the scholar he could now ask his questions. The scholar remained silent, as he no longer had anything to ask.

DON'T TRY

Poet Charles Bukowski has the words "don't try" written on his tombstone. *Star Wars* fans will remember Yoda's famous advice to Luke Skywalker, "Do or do not. There is no try."

These maxims can be confusing to many people, as they're diametrically opposed to Western culture's emphasis on goals and outcomes. We are taught from childhood that winning is the most important thing in the world and that happiness comes only from achievements. Ironically, the most "successful" people in the world are often prone to depression, drug addiction or worse. We see it with professional athletes, Hollywood actors and Wall Street business executives; all the success in the world cannot fill the void one feels inside when material goods and ego-driven achievements are the only motivation in life.

When Bukowski says don't try, he doesn't mean that you should give up on life and sit on the couch all day watching YouTube videos while you stuff your face full of gluten free snack cakes. Yoda and Bukowski were both trying to convey the Buddhist concept sometimes called "effortless effort"—the idea that letting go of an attachment to any outcome frees you up and allows you to be fully present in the moment. When we forget the goal, we have no choice but to focus on the process itself. If you are always focused on goals, you will miss the entire journey. Instead, focus on doing each little task along the way with care and attention. Get lost in the moment; it is the only path to true joy.

The specifics of training don't matter if you don't take action. Three sets of ten? Two sets of twenty? You can have the best plan on paper, but it means nothing until you actually do it.

PUMPING IRONY

I realize there's inherent irony in writing about how talk is cheap. Though the written word tends to have more of an authoritative feel to it than speech (where do you think the word "author" comes from?), reading can't do much more to help you take action than talking can. In fact, I have a confession to make: The Kavadlo Brothers can't really improve your life. Only you can do that. Nobody outside of you can ever affect change in your life. Not us or anyone else. You and only you—and that's the only way it's ever going to be.

That's right, nothing outside of yourself can ever bring you happiness or fulfillment, but maybe these words can help you come to that realization.

Let this book be the finger that points you to the moon. But please, don't miss that heavenly glory!

THE SUNK COST FALLACY

—BY DANNY KAVADLO

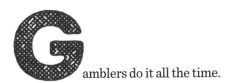

Author's Insight—

I wanted to paint a picture of desperation here because so many people feel fear and misery when it comes to starting a fitness program. But ultimately, the sentiment of my musings is positive, as this terror is generally unfounded. The decisions you make now are the ones that matter. We often grow attached to things—not only possessions, but also lifestyles and habits. We find it hard to change... but it doesn't have to be. You are always you, and you are always in the present. If not now, when?

Gamblers do it all the time.

You've seen them in Vegas. Atlantic City. New Orleans. They're pumping money into shiny machines, stacking chips on velvet-covered tables, spinning their wheels at roulette. With tired eyes squinting through the thick, blue smoke, they see a fantastical vision of recovering what they've lost. In all likelihood, they won't.

I imagine the thought process goes something like this: You've lost thousands and are continuing on a downward spiral, but you've already spent so much that *this time*, you gotta win! You're due for a little luck anyhow. How could you not hit? You think that if you just keep at it, you will get back at least the cost you invested, maybe even a little more. But this is a fallacy. The cost is lost, my friend. Zed's dead, baby.

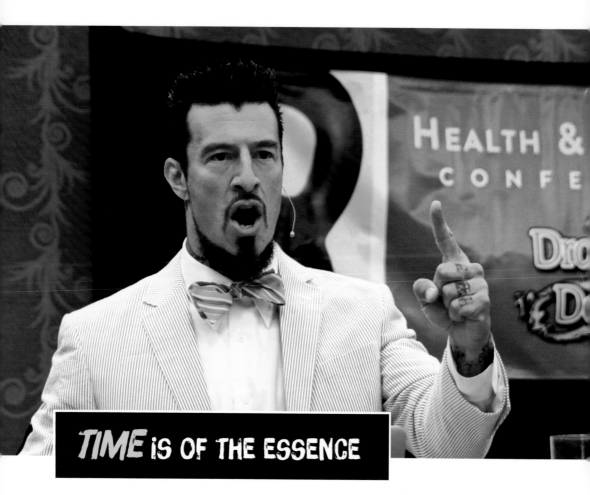

TIME is OF THE ESSENCE

It's why people hold onto falling stocks, hoping for a rebound, or spend all day at the track with nothing to show, rather than cutting their losses. Ultimately, you must do something different because what you're doing isn't working.

Sadly, money is not the only investment in which so many double down after losing. There are numerous others. Time immediately comes to mind, and it's a far more worthy commodity than cash. You're stuck at a dead end job. You hate it, but you've been there forever. "Oh, I can't leave," you say meekly to yourself. "It's too late to go anywhere else. I've already invested so much time."

So what?

You won't get that time back, even if you stay. Don't focus on your diminishing returns. Just leave. If you think it's too late to start something else and change your behavior and life, then we have a major problem on our hands. As the saying goes, *time is of the essence*. You go now!

Yet even more valuable than time and money is love. Yes, our most wondrous emotion (or oftentimes, a lack of it) has been known to fall victim to the sunk cost fallacy as well. Have you ever been in a toxic relationship that lasted way longer than it should? Have you ever grown so accustomed to another's smile that it no longer brings you joy, only pain? Or even worse, indifference? Have you ever held on, when there remains nothing worthwhile to cling to? I reckon we all have, and I'm sorry if you've suffered. Each one of us lives in pain at times, but if you're stuck in a situation like this, you gotta get the hell out. That's all I got to say about that.

All of these scenarios involve protecting yourself *from yourself.* No one can love another if they cannot love themselves. Yes, I'm telling you to love yourself wholly: emotionally, spiritually and personally.

The great thing about nurturing your own physical body is that (barring injury or disability) it's the one thing over which you have complete control. There is a direct correlation between effort and yield. Your body isn't a slot machine; there is no need for luck here. No matter how many hours you spend at the casino, it does not guarantee success. But putting hours into your training does!

For that matter, you can write the world's greatest song, but if it doesn't sell, you will have little or no validation of your craft. You can paint an amazing portrait, but if no one buys it, your career as an artist will not prosper. This is not the case with fitness. If you make a change today, and remain consistent, it will show. It is not contingent on anything outside of yourself. That's part of what makes working out so real and beautiful. It's the only phenomenon in this world where you truly reap what you sow.

Don't subscribe to the sunk cost fallacy when it comes to your own being. So what if you haven't trained in a week or a year or since high school? Try not to look at the sunk cost behind you. Look at what can be in front of you instead. It's not too late to start a personal revolution today. Don't gamble with your health.

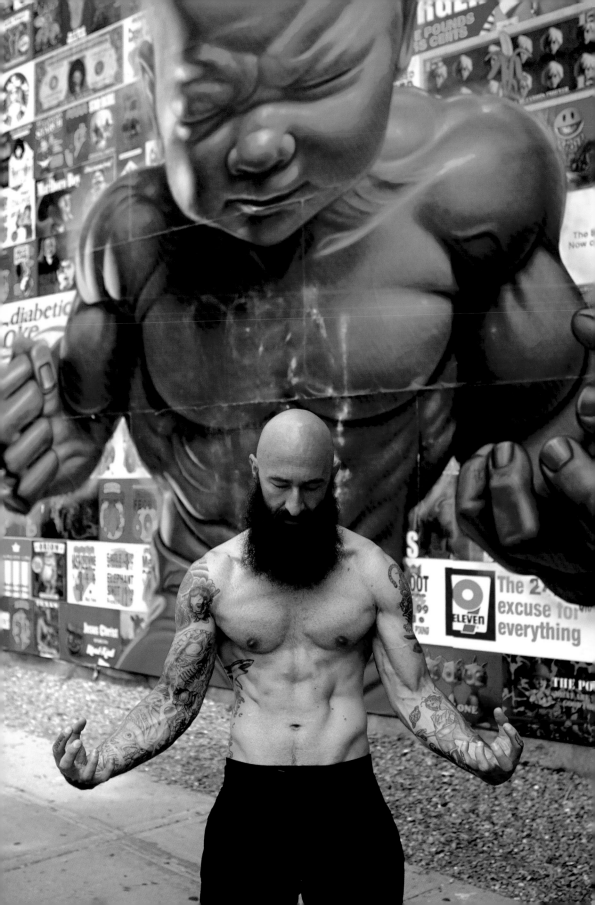

STRENGTH
FROM WITHIN

—BY AL KAVADLO

Author's Insight—

This piece was originally published on Bodybuilding.com in April of 2013 with the title "Your Hidden Source Of Strength: 3 Steps To Better Breathing." It's not uncommon for an editor to change the title of an article to make it more clickable on the web. I didn't quite feel like the "3 steps" concept worked for this piece, however, so I've changed the title back to one I feel is more appropriate.

All of the most powerful entities in the universe source their energy from the inside out. The Earth relies on its core heat to maintain a surface temperature warm enough to sustain life. A volcano is calm on the surface but the lava below could wipe out every living creature for miles, should it erupt. When an atomic bomb is detonated, the explosion starts in the center and expands. And if you ever want to do a one arm push-up, one leg squat or any other high-level calisthenics exercise, you'll need to learn to tap into your deep internal forces, too.

When performing a push-up, your chest, triceps and shoulders are doing the bulk of the work, but your lats, traps and rhomboids must act as stabilizers for you to maintain proper form. Your glutes, lower back and abs also need to work together to keep the body straight. You might not notice how much your entire body is involved in a basic move like a push-up, but if you want to perform a *one arm* push-up, you're going to need to use every muscle in your entire body. And that starts from the inside out—with your breath.

BREATHE RIGHT

It may sound ridiculous, but most people don't really know how to breathe. Yes, your reptilian brain is smart enough to get enough air in your lungs to keep you alive, but when was the last time you really filled them to capacity? How about emptied them completely? There is a world of power in the breath! Learn to harness it, and you'll be one step closer to bodyweight mastery.

Everyone knows the abs are a crucial part of core strength and most are aware of the role of strong obliques. Clever trainers will also point out the importance of the lower back muscles in overall core strength, as they act as an antagonist to the abdominals. However, there is another antagonist to the abs that most people overlook which also plays a crucial role in core strength: the diaphragm.

Your diaphragm is a powerful muscle inside your belly that controls your breath; it's arguably the single most important muscle in your body, after your heart. During inhalation, the diaphragm contracts, creating space for your lungs to expand. When you breathe out, the diaphragm relaxes.

Go ahead and take a big breath right now. Did your chest rise? It shouldn't. Proper activation of the diaphragm draws the breath deep into the belly.

If you're having a hard time figuring out how to breathe into your belly, try lying on your back or standing upright with one hand on your abdomen, then take a deep breath, trying to expand your belly against your hand. It may take some trial and error to figure out, so if your chest or shoulders rise, breathe out and try again. This will come easier for some than others—it may be very different than what you're accustomed to.

Eventually you should be able to take a big breath into your belly without your chest or shoulders moving at all. Once you've figured out how to do that, the next step is to exhale while deeply contracting your core from the inside. You can gradually let air seep out as you tighten your abdominal contraction. There is an opening inside your throat called the glottis that you can use to block air from exiting your lungs, like a built-in pressure valve. Practicing this technique will help you learn to control your breath and use your diaphragm and glottis to tense your body from the inside out.

STATIC ELECTRICITY

Total body tension is often easiest to learn by practicing static holds. Try using the breathing technique we just practiced during an isometric plank. Get onto your elbows and toes with your body in a straight line from the back of your head to your heels. Focus on your breath and begin squeezing your whole body as you exhale: abs, glutes, inner thighs, quads—everything. The more you tense your entire body, the less any one part has to shoulder the burden. Once you get the feel for creating total body tension, you'll soon be ready to transfer that newfound power to harder moves like the L-sit, for example.

WAITING TO EXHALE

Breath control is great for static holds but it's also beneficial when practicing difficult dynamic exercises—particularly the one arm push-up or one leg squat. The valsalva maneuver is a breathing technique that's well-known in powerlifting circles, though it can be useful in bodyweight training as well. The technique involves using your diaphragm to create a bubble of air in your belly to stabilize the trunk during heavy lifting. As you have to hold your breath while you do it, the technique is often discouraged by fitness professionals. In fact, the first time I ever saw the term "valsalva maneuver" was in a personal training textbook warning about the dangers of using the technique for barbell training.

The truth is, lots of lifters have had great success with the valsalva maneuver. Though there is a slight risk of fainting when using the technique during a heavy lift (particularly if you have a history of fainting and/or high blood pressure), I've never seen anyone pass out during a one leg bodyweight squat. I've seen people fall on their butt, but I haven't seen a single one lose consciousness.

To use the valsalva maneuver during a one arm push-up or one leg squat, inhale into your belly during the lowering phase of the movement, then hold your breath briefly at the bottom and keep it there as you begin coming up. Wait to exhale until you are just shy of halfway up—the "sticking point" as it's often known. The air bubble in your belly will help stabilize your spine during this critical transition point. The breath need not be held more than a second or two for each rep—any longer could have adverse effects. Additionally, as doing many consecutive reps in this manner may rapidly increase your blood pressure, the valsalva technique works best when applied to low rep ranges.

Though learning to control your breath can help you tap into your total body strength, there's no magic bullet in the world of fitness. These techniques can help, but there will never be any way to achieve advanced bodyweight feats without commitment and effort. It takes practice to advance in calisthenics, but if you put in the time and get to know your body, it's a journey worth taking. Pay attention to your breath; you may be surprised by how much it can teach you.

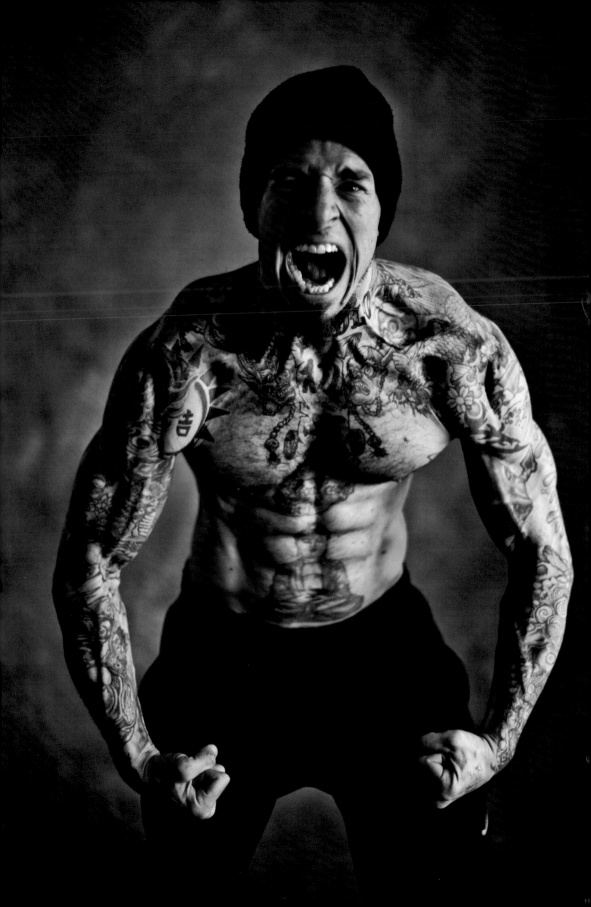

THE CALISTHENICS BODY

—BY DANNY KAVADLO

> ### Author's Insight—
>
> This piece was initially intended to be a commercial of sorts for calisthenics. I wanted to focus on the visual attraction that so many people have toward the physique that results from bodyweight strength training. I also sought to dispel the misconception that there is something wrong with training for aesthetics. All fitness goals are virtuous pursuits, and I was tired of the "functional fitness police" asserting the notion that training for looks is a bad thing. But as I sat down to compose this article, I realized that there was even more that I wanted to say.
>
> I am very pleased that calisthenics has been gaining more notoriety in the commercial fitness world, but I noticed some people in the media who were acting like they invented it. I am often leery of internet boasts. For the record, calisthenics predates every other form of strength training and no one individual conceived it. While always refreshing and inspiring, calisthenics isn't new. The final article became my most popular to date.

Lately, there's been a lot written about calisthenic strength training. Calisthenics—or bodyweight—training is hotter than ever. Ironically, a modality that's existed since the dawn of man is being talked about like it's a brand new phenomenon. Before the invention of treadmills, barbells and cable crossovers, mankind was getting strong and ripped using nothing more for resistance than our own bodies. Pressing, pulling and squatting are hard-wired into our DNA. So why all the hoopla about calisthenics? Why now?

Some claim it's the trend toward minimalism. Others say it's the feeling of empowerment you get from owning a body that's truly self-made. Perhaps others are impressed by the many feats of strength associated with extreme calisthenics. I actually think all of these answers are right, but there's something more, too.

Let's face it. Everybody who works out pays attention to aesthetics to some degree. No matter how "functional" or "sport specific" one's training may be, we all react to imagery. What has become known as the Calisthenics Body is easily identifiable by a rippled, muscular physique, erect posture and no superfluous body fat. Say what you will: *That's* what really gets people talking!

One of the beautiful things about calisthenics is that we celebrate the use of our whole body cohesively, rather than attempting to isolate small body parts one-at-a-time. And while there is no doubt that different exercises emphasize certain muscles more than others, I'd like to be clear that 100% isolation in any modality is impossible.

The principles of calisthenic strength training have a direct physical manifestation because the strength to weight ratio required has specific demands. Practitioners of calisthenics develop that ideal balance of muscle mass and body fat that allows for dominance of their realm. The body doesn't lie. There are telltale signs.

ABS

In calisthenics training, bar-work is often emphasized for abs. Exercises such as hanging leg raises have a direct effect on the abs' overall appearance. One of the reasons is that in addition to the abdominal muscles, these exercises rely heavily on the serratus anterior (which is not generally considered an abs muscle) for stability. This has a huge effect by shaping and framing the entire abdominal region. A ripped serratus, and the bulging six-pack abs contained within, are the markings of the Calisthenics Body.

Furthermore, when you train calisthenics, you use your abs for every single exercise and it shows!

ARMS

The unmistakable horseshoe shaped triceps and oversized baseball biceps are a signature sign of the Calisthenics Body. The pronounced "peak" is further enhanced by the popping, powerhouse deltoids.

It can take any number of machine-based isolation style exercises to hit the arms (and chest and shoulders) from as many angles as the good old-fashioned push-up. Performed deep, with full range of motion, the results are undeniable. They can also be done on a multitude of surfaces and inclines. Have some fun!

Just as with abs, bar-work can be your best friend when it comes to arms, particularly biceps, which get a better workout from chin-ups than from all the curls in the world. Because you're pulling far more weight than you would typically curl, the gains are astronomical. Chin-ups (or "pull-ups" as the overhand version is known) and their many variations create amazing tensile strength and powerful connective tissue. Combine the grip training you get from bar-work with advanced push-up variations for forearms that would make Popeye jealous.

BACK/SHOULDERS/CHEST

Exceptionally wide lats are a trademark of the Calisthenics Body. Because we don't attempt to isolate the arms, we have a greater chance of unlocking the genetic potential of our lats through pull-ups. The upper frame associated with calisthenics is said to be that perfect "V-shape" and the lats play a huge role. Wide lats and strong posture are a direct result of a progressive bodyweight pulling program. The shoulders cap it off.

Your shoulders are used in all upper body calisthenics strength training and get a substantial workout from every exercise mentioned thus far. The "V" gets even wider when we train handstand push-ups. Even folks who think they can military press massive poundage are often humbled when they attempt this exercise. Handstand push-ups lead to huge gains in the shoulders. Take 'em slow and controlled. Touch your nose to the ground.

Of course, the push-up is the granddaddy of all chest exercises. The classic we all learned in gym class is a spectacular exercise in its own right. But beyond that, we can play with inclines, limit points of contact or increase range of motion. All of these methods employ progressive techniques to build a thick, hard, powerful chest. A great example of this is the feet elevated push-up, which is guaranteed to send your pecs into maximum overdrive!

LEGS

When you train your legs using only your bodyweight, they get strong! Not from external resistance, but rather from manipulating gravity and doing complete movement patterns. Bodyweight squats go all the way to the ground—ass to ankles. I'm more concerned with building strength through the full expression of a movement than from overloaded half-reps where the hamstrings never touch the calf. Try doing forty bodyweight squats all the way down. If that sounds easy, try doing five... on just one leg!

Exercises like single leg squats also enhance our inborn balance. We push, pull and stabilize from all our leg muscles, in a perfect marriage of strength and mobility. Additionally, bridging exercises require further recruitment of the hamstrings, calves and glutes. Raw strength and supreme flexibility are the markings of a bodyweight warrior's legs.

Critics of calisthenics sometimes perpetuate the falsehood that bodyweight athletes have underdeveloped legs. Ironically these are the same unfounded jabs that have rocked the weightlifting community for years. There are many ways to skin a cat, and we all have more in common than apart. No matter how you choose to work out, everybody's legs need training!

CONFIDENCE

This one is harder to quantify than the others, but you know it when you see it. Any red-blooded man or woman who's sure they could pull their body up to (or over) a bar, conducts themselves with a certain quiet cool that cannot be explained. The posture and physique is unmistakable. When you know your own pound-for pound power and truly own the Calisthenics Body, you stand tall!

A Few Of My Favorite Things

—By Danny Kavadlo

Author's Insight—

I wrote the original version of this article on the Progressive Calisthenics Certification blog in 2013, and it's amazing to me how well it's held up. I wanted to get away from discussing specific exercises and talk about the bond we have with our environment when we train. We all need a place to call home. Years later, all of these places are still a few of my favorite things!

Something I cherish about calisthenics is that you can do it anywhere. That fact in itself is endlessly fascinating to me. In a day and age where people sit in traffic while they drive to the gym, or wait an hour in line to take a 30-minute spin class on a fake bike, the simple notion that a gym isn't necessary is truly liberating.

Now, please understand that I have nothing against the gym. It can be a great place to train. I have had many spectacular workouts in gyms. I just believe that the gym is not the only game in town. Due to the simple and sublime nature of bodyweight strength training, you can make a gym out of almost any place you want. That's one of my favorite things.

These places themselves are a few of my favorite things, too.

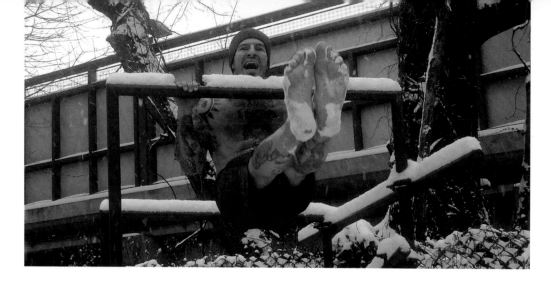

IN THE BACKYARD

Several years ago it dawned on me that the ultimate home gym could be mine, but I'd have to build it. So for a low price, plus some time and sweat, I built my first backyard pull-up bar. I could now rip through those reps anytime the urge struck me. This was even better than the indoor, mounted bars I've owned for most of my life. You see, I have always been a fan of outdoor workouts. I love being outside in general—the feel of the ground beneath my toes, the wind in my hair and the taste of the air on my lips gives me a physical sensation that makes me feel truly alive. Sadly these days, it seems we have a cultural obsession with climate control. We drive in cars with individually heated seats and exercise in air-conditioned buildings. I am pleased to say that the outdoor workout eliminates those unnecessary commodities. Nowhere can you dominate your own bodyweight and release your inner beast like you can under the Earth's sky, alone with the elements, rain, shine or snow, in touch with who you are.

At any time of day, any time of year, all my favorite exercises are waiting at my doorstep. From perfect planks to powerful pull-ups, they're all here. It is also of note that these iron bars have a big, fat two-inch diameter, which adds extreme grip training to every single workout. We train hard in Brooklyn!

IN THE PARK

I am lucky enough to live in New York City, one of the main hubs for bodyweight enthusiasts from all walks of life. There are many parks, playgrounds and jungle gyms in the Big Apple, but none are as well known throughout the world as Alphabet City's legendary Tompkins Square Park.

I've trained a hundred times at TSP at six o'clock on a Monday morning. While the city sleeps, serious-minded individuals can be found lunging, jumping, pushing and pulling.

Even in the rain or snow, you can always find some hardcore bodyweight aficionados out there doing their thing. In fact, it's the first place I ever saw a one-arm pull-up.

But just as it is motivational to train amongst those serious athletes, it moves me equally to see how many newcomers train at TSP as well. You see, a certain solidarity exists at Tompkins. It spans across the entire community of the park, from the world-renowned bar masters, all the way down to the young kids doing their first chin-up. Where else could you observe an ex-con asking a drag queen for handstand advice? I've seen it at Tompkins. Ya' gotta love Alphabet City!

IN THE BASEMENT

Sometimes I train indoors. Remember, by keeping things simple and pure, based on mechanics and movement, we can train anywhere we want to. So do push-ups in your kitchen. Practice your bridge in the living room. Put a pull-up bar in the hallway. I personally like to train in the basement.

The basement has been used as a metaphor for the subconscious by everybody from Dostoevsky to the cult classic television series "Wilfred." And it makes sense. When we are in the basement, we are in the building's underground, free to explore the deepest, most primordial workings of its structure... and of our own.

Much of calisthenics training is based on unleashing our instinctual, primordial movement patterns. Arguably, all forms of bar-work tap into your "tree dwelling" DNA as you pull your own bodyweight from a hanging position when executing pull-ups, muscle-ups and more. Furthermore, the deep down, full range of motion squat, where the back of the thigh comes in full contact with the calf is so primitive that both monkeys and children do it on a regular basis. You don't get more ancient than that.

There is no better place to explore the deep, dark movements of the mind, spirit, and body than underground, with just your physical self and your psyche.

IN THE END

These places are just a few of my favorite things. Hopefully you have discovered some special workout spots that are near and dear to you. We all need somewhere we can work on self-improvement and awareness. Explore your options and be creative. Have fun with it. And as always, keep the dream alive!

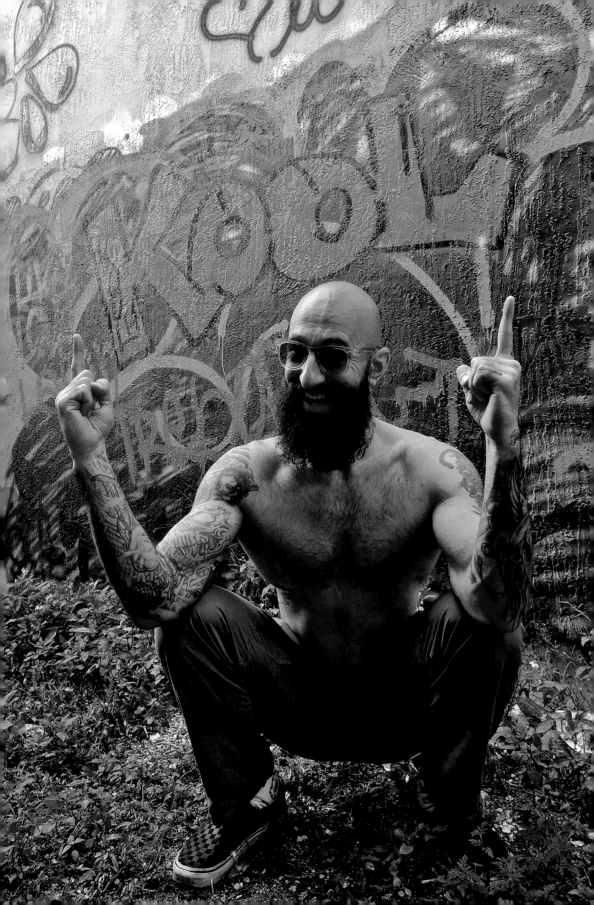

Squats Happening

—BY AL KAVADLO

 uring a recent workout at my local park, I observed a father and son playing a game of catch. The dad was around my age and the boy looked to be about three years old.

At one point the child missed the ball and the dad went to retrieve it. I watched him bend down with his back rounded, shoulders slumped and knees pitched way over his feet. What you might call "bad form" on a squat.

A few minutes later, the boy missed the ball again, but this time the father let him retrieve it himself. When the tot picked up the ball, he squatted down from his hips with his chest tall and lifted it without the slightest bend in his back—or any overt awareness of the movement pattern. It seemed to happen very naturally. He certainly had no idea that what he'd just done can be difficult for most of my beginning personal training clients.

Squatting is one of the human body's most fundamental movement patterns, yet through years of neglect, many adults have forgotten something that once came effortlessly. Children instinctively perform perfect squats, yet most adults have spent our lives sitting in couches, chairs and cars, steering our bodies away from natural squatting. We've done this to the point where we've unlearned instinctive habits like lifting from the legs, and replaced them with lower back pain and hip ailments. Though we live in a world where most people spend almost all their waking hours in some sort of chair, it is not too late for you to relearn this primal movement pattern.

HOW LOW CAN YOU GO?

Relearning a full bodyweight squat may be a more formidable task for some than others. Newcomers and people with limited mobility might not be able to get very deep into a squat without sacrificing their form. This is to be expected, but let's set some boundaries of what constitutes a proper squat. I don't mind if your knees track forward, but we always want to be sure that our heels are flat during squats, with weight evenly distributed throughout the feet and toes. It's okay to allow yourself some degree of forward bending in the bottom of a bodyweight squat when you're working on mobility. In time, the plan should be to eventually squat ass-to-ankles with a tall chest and straight back for the entire range of motion, but until that's possible, just try to stay as upright as you can.

If you are having a hard time keeping your heels down, I suggest holding onto a doorframe or other sturdy object for support. Hold on tight, but keep your shoulders relaxed as you sit back onto your heels, sinking down as deep as you can. While keeping your heels planted, think about flexing your ankles so your knees track forward in line with your toes. Eventually, you will learn to rely less on the support of the object and begin to find the bottom of the squat on your own.

HOLD IT RIGHT THERE

I recommend spending some time in the bottom position of a squat every day to help restore a full range of motion. The benefits of holding this position include increased hip mobility, increased ankle mobility, improved spinal health, improved knee health and of course, improved technique on your squats, so you can make your legs powerful and capable through a full range of motion.

Remember, when starting out you may need to grab onto a sturdy object for balance. You'll likely feel a big stretch in your hips, groin and calves. This is good. Take a deep breath and try to relax into it. Start out by holding this position for one minute and gradually work up to holds of several minutes or longer.

HIPS, HIPS, HOORAY!

After practicing for a few days or weeks, you should begin to feel more comfortable holding the bottom of a squat. Eventually this can become a resting position that you'll be able to stay in for extended periods of time. In some cultures, this is what people do instead of sitting in chairs.

One more thing you can try when you're down there holding your deep squat is to place your hands in a prayer position in front of your chest, with your elbows against the insides of your knees, in order to leverage them open for a deeper hip stretch. Again, breathe deep and try to relax into the stretch.

If you feel like practicing these holds on a daily basis may be too much for you, start out doing them every other day and eventually work toward a daily practice. In time, you may even find yourself resting in a squat, instead of a chair.

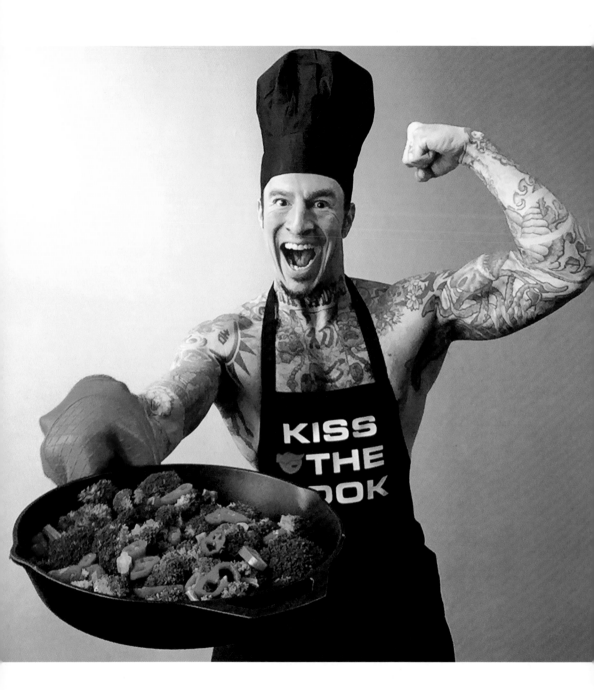

GET STRONG

Six Tips For A Six Pack

—By Danny Kavadlo

Author's Insight—

This article appeared in its original form in 2014 on Bodybuilding.com. It was written as a tie-in to my second Dragon Door title, Diamond-Cut Abs. DCA was the abs book I always wished I had as a kid, and my first book to achieve Amazon Bestseller status. What I believe made this book so successful was that it focused on what you put into your body as much (or even more) as what you do with it. For that reason, I made an executive decision not to include any tips on exercise in this article. Followers of the Get Strong program will have questions about diet. This piece provides insight into the Kavadlo approach to nutrition.

There's no denying that abs are a core component of perceived physical beauty (pun intended). Almost every magazine cover, advertisement and billboard shows images of chiseled abs. "Ideal" waistlines have gotten smaller and smaller over the years, as we as a culture continue to celebrate abs more than ever. Love it or hate it, such is the world. In fact, I'd say that just about anyone who has ever worked out in any capacity has at one point or another—even if they won't admit it today—focused specifically on their abs. Why?

Because abdominal strength is important: You use your abs every time you lift, twist or even stand up. I'm not just talking about aesthetics here (although that is a fine motivation as well). A powerful set of abs, along with a strong, balanced physique is part of the formula for overall physical health. Still, one fact cannot be ignored: You can't train your way out of a poor diet. It's a cliché because it's true.

While there is an extraordinary amount of conflicting testimony regarding proper nutrition, there are a few broad strokes on which we can all agree. Some are both mind-blowing and obvious at the same time.

FIRE IT UP

First things first, we need to be aware of what we're eating. The best way to do this is to prepare as many of your own meals as possible. When you cook for yourself, you know exactly what every single ingredient is, not to mention how much was used in preparation. When consuming foods made by others, you really don't know much for certain, particularly when dining out. Many times, even when prepared by "healthy" restaurants, meals are laden with gratuitous amounts of grease, salt and chemicals. These meals are often served to you in oversized portions. I've seen dishes labeled as salads and sides that could make even the most active of individuals gain weight.

When making your meals, keep your ingredients few and simple. Use whole ingredients and avoid packaged foods; their labels are often misleading. Health claims like "fat free," "no sugar" and "low carb" (to name just a few) are written by marketing honchos, whose job is to generate revenue, not to make you lean. In reality, the best foods, like vegetables, fruits, nuts and quality meats, don't come in a printed package.

Despite what is frequently perpetrated, paying attention to eating whole, locally sourced and minimally processed foods is easier and tastier than people think. And guess what? If you eat good foods most of the time, there is nothing you will have to avoid all of the time.

GO GREEN

A lot of folks think I eat nothing but pull-up bars and tattoos. They'd be surprised to see how many leafy greens I consume. Everyone knows that green vegetables are an excellent source of vitamins, nutrients and dietary fiber, but many don't realize what a large role eating foods like spinach, kale and broccoli can have in sculpting amazing abs.

In my youth, it took me many years of experimentation to find out which eating styles work best for me, not just in terms of abs, but in terms of life. Many so-called experts go out of their way to complicate things, often referring to the components of foods rather than the foods themselves. I do not believe that making things sound complicated makes them any more valid. Actually, I've observed the opposite to be true. Obsessively measuring macros, antioxidants or even calories does not necessarily lead to results. Sure, it is very fine to have some idea of how much you're consuming, but stressing out over minute details will often get you nowhere. Let's use common sense instead. We know that spinach is good for you. We know that cupcakes (even organic ones) can lead to weight gain.

Greens, like most vegetables, are extremely low in calories. No need to overthink; this is common knowledge. Those who have problems with self-control and portion size really can't go wrong when it comes to greens, which can be consumed virtually whenever you want, in as large of a portion as you desire. (Just don't smother them in ranch dressing or decadent amounts of oil.) I recommend loading two thirds of your dinner plate with veggies. This will keep you filled with quality nutrition and may prevent you from making some sketchier choices, which brings me to my next point.

AVOID PROCESSED SUGAR

Again, let's keep it simple. If you consume extra sugar and do not metabolize it quickly, it will be stored as fat. Many of us tend to store this fat on our bellies. Clearly, a diet high in sugar will hinder your mission toward six-pack abs.

In fact, processed sugar is among your abs' greatest foes. By this, I am not just referring to white table sugar and high fructose corn syrup, but to just about any product where everything has been removed but the sugar. This includes "raw" and "natural" sugars, as well as "nectars," "beet sugar" and many other misleadingly labeled sweeteners on the market.

The natural sugars found in fruits and vegetables do not fall into this category, as they have never been processed or stripped of their natural fiber. They are therefore metabolized slowly over time. An apple is not only sweet, it's filling and free of processed sugar, making it a great snack for ultimate abs.

DRINK MORE WATER

One of the worst things about the aforementioned sugar is that it is added to virtually everything. While it's obvious that beverages like fruity cocktails and syrupy sodas will stand in our way on the quest for abs, many well-intentioned individuals still drink their sugar unknowingly in the form of flavored waters, sweetened iced teas, fruit juices and more. These products should be consumed minimally, if at all. I urge you to look at ingredients and nutritional information. Things are not always what they seem. A glass of orange juice has over 100 calories and 20 grams of sugar. Water has none. The importance of drinking good old H2O cannot be overstated.

Water improves metabolic rate and digestion, which helps you get leaner. It hydrates and moisturizes, thus increasing your skin's suppleness. Water also fills you up, making it less likely for you to snack on unsavory choices. Furthermore, water removes toxins and reduces aches and pains, helping you train harder and recover faster.

EAT LESS

I will be the first to acknowledge that there are many paths one can take toward achieving ultimate abs. Lots of eating styles have the potential to help you get lean. Although there is no weight-loss method universally proven to work perfectly for everyone in all situations, simply eating less comes pretty close!

Having a ripped six pack requires having a low body fat percentage (10% or less for men, 20% or less for women). If you are carrying extra mass on your midsection, you will need to metabolize it. Keeping your stomach perpetually full will prevent this from happening.

In other words, if you want to show off that hard-earned definition, you may have to eat less. You can survive on fewer calories than you think.

LIVE LIFE

When eating for abs, it's important to show restraint, not deprivation. A system that leaves you constantly wanting more will inevitably leave you dissatisfied. Long term deprivation can lead to a backlash of bad habits, and is often counterproductive in the long run. I think it's best to have a healthful, holistic approach to training and nutrition. Look at the big picture. Food is meant to be enjoyed.

For that matter, life is also meant to be enjoyed. This is why I recommend making broad lifestyle changes rather than rote dieting. No eating style, program or fitness goal should take away from the fulfillment you feel from doing the things you love. Have fun, see the world, spend time with people you care about.

When all is said and done, each of us is a product of our own day-to-day habits. If you eat well 80-90% of the time, there is no reason you cannot indulge the remaining 10-20%. In fact, I *encourage it!* This principle is true for desserts, cheat meals and celebratory dinners, all of which are fine because they are occasional. Just make sure to be honest and hold yourself accountable; a "cheat" is not an exception if you do it every day.

If you have good eating habits, there's almost nothing you'll have to avoid 100% of the time, leaving you and your six-pack abs free to live your life.

I'm Walking Here!

—By Al Kavadlo

Author's Insight—

Inspiration sometimes comes from unexpected sources. In the summer of 2015, Danny, my wife Grace and I had the pleasure of working with photographer Neil Gavin, who had an idea to take a very simple photo of the three of us walking down the street. When he suggested the photo, I didn't really get what he was going for. However, when I saw the image later on, I instantly loved it. In fact, it inspired me to write this piece about how much I enjoy a good walk.

In my book Zen Mind, Strong Body, there is a chapter entitled, "Is Walking Really the Best Exercise?" My conclusion there was that, contrary to conventional wisdom, walking is not the best form of exercise: Strength training is. While I stand by that assertion, you shouldn't dismiss the many benefits of walking either. This piece can be seen as a counterpoint to that one, as it extolls those benefits.

We've all been there: It's the day after a brutal leg workout, and all you want to do is sit on your butt and rest. Your thighs hurt, your calves feel stiff and your lower back moans at even the thought of standing. I, too, have fallen into this trap. Sitting feels good when you're sore, and initiating movement can be unpleasant at first. However, once you get going, an hour or two of low-intensity activity is known to aid your body in achieving optimal recovery. So what's the best choice? Treadmill? Stationary bike? Nope—for me, it's walking.

Moving your legs can help prevent muscular soreness from increasing in the days following an intense leg workout, and maybe even help to eliminate it entirely. Getting your blood flowing can also be helpful for reducing inflammation and stiffness. Going for a stroll is a fantastic way to promote circulation, particularly in your lower body. Where do you think the expression "walk it off" comes from?

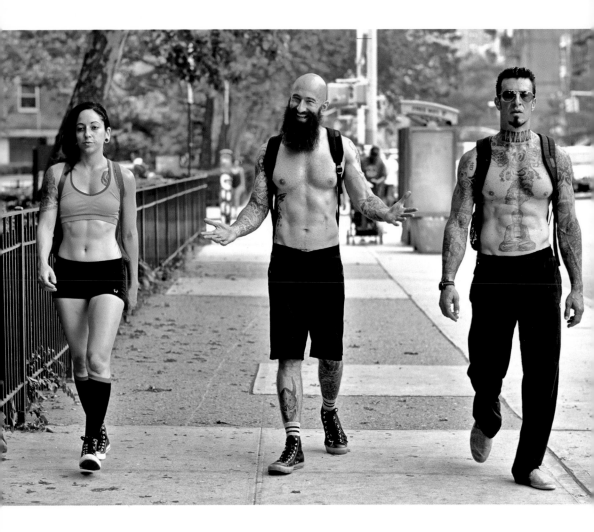

An hour or two of walking can also add up in terms of caloric output, which is a nice benefit if you're the type of person who abhors cardio. Add a steep enough incline into the mix and the cardiovascular benefits of walking can begin to increase exponentially.

If you live in a metropolitan area (or have a short commute) you can use walking as a mode of transportation. As a New York City resident, I walk for an hour or more every day just to run errands and get around town, but I still make time for additional walks simply for their own sake. Walking makes sense for getting around in a busy city, but no matter where you live, it's worth going for a long walk a few times a week (in addition to your strength training, of course).

Besides the physical benefits, walking can be an excellent way to relieve stress. That phrase "walk it off" can apply to more than just sore legs; If I'm upset about something, a long walk can often help me simmer down and deal with pent up frustrations. A solitary stroll can be a calming, meditative experience. In this day and age, we rarely get to spend time alone with our thoughts, though that is often what many of us need. It's nice to have the chance to think things through without the distractions that inevitably come up at home or in the office. Though the first few minutes may feel tedious, the longer I walk for, the more quickly time seems to pass.

If you're being mindful, you can learn a lot about your body mechanics by paying attention to your gait. You can even use walking to gauge your posture and screen your movement quality.

Ask yourself the following questions during your walk to assess yourself:

✔ Are your footfalls light and airy, or heavy and lumbering?

✔ Do your feet maintain their integrity throughout each phase of your stride, or do your arches collapse as you transition from your heel to your forefoot?

✔ Is your chest tall with your shoulders relaxed, or are you hunched over?

As you go through that checklist, make it a point to correct and improve whatever you can. If you notice yourself crashing down hard on your heels, focus on controlling your steps and landing more gently. If your arches are collapsing, think about engaging your ankle and toe muscles to bring stability to your stride. If your posture is problematic, imagine a string is attached to the top of your head, then pretend that you are being pulled upward by that string. Ideally, your shoulders should wind up above your hips, rather than in front of them or behind them. Focus on looking ahead, rather than down, as looking down can negatively affect your posture as well.

In addition to being a great way to enjoy some time alone, walking can also be a relaxing way to spend leisure time with friends and family. If you've got a sedentary loved one who you've been trying to help inspire toward fitness, a long walk on a nice day is a great way to introduce them to a healthier lifestyle without the impending anxiety that a formal workout can produce. If you are a dog lover, bring your furry friends along for the journey. Pets needs exercise, too!

While walking on its own is certainly not enough to get anyone in shape, it's a nice addition to a balanced training program with many benefits, as well as a worthwhile activity in its own right.

So what are you waiting for? Let's get to walk!

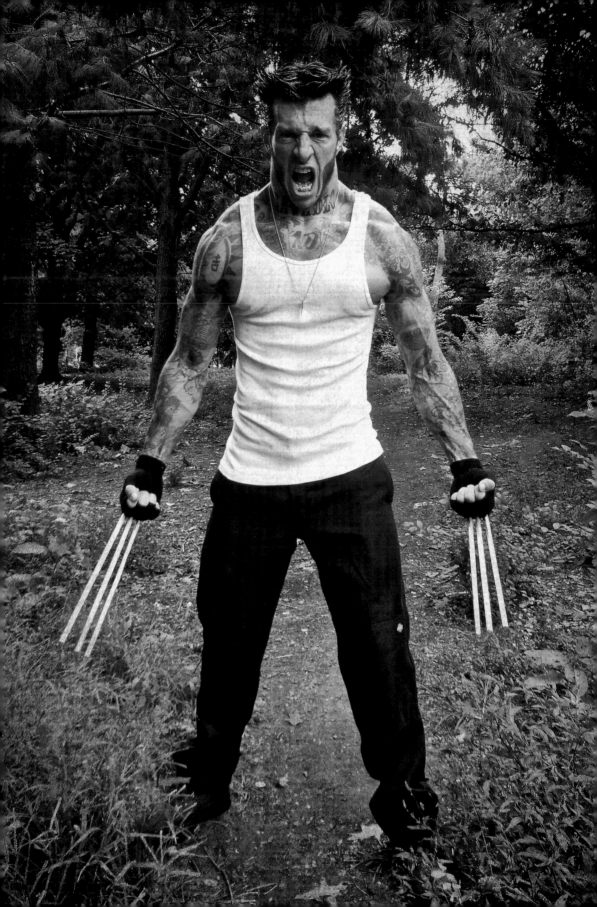

Healing Powers

—By Danny Kavadlo

Author's Insight—

I wrote "Healing Powers" for Dragon Door's Progressive Calisthenics Certification Blog in March of 2015. I had recently read an article from a very popular source that spoke so much about potential training injuries that it almost discouraged exercise. Sure, anyone who trains may get an occasional nick or ding from time to time. This happens to people who don't train, too. I felt compelled to express that working out is healthier and safer than not working out. Plus, I love superhero tie-ins!

Wouldn't it be great if we all had healing powers? Think about it. If the perils of injury were non-existent? If the chances of maiming, straining or spraining any particular body part were a work of fiction, best suited for the comic books? What if the words "pain" and "gain" were not so frequently associated?

Marvel at a universe where getting hurt is not a major concern.

Well here's the thing, bub: It's NOT a major concern. Not much of one anyway. Now before you start freaking out, try hearing me out. Yes, I acknowledge that it is possible that one can get injured doing a pull-up (or lifting weights, running, jumping, walking down the street, etc.) But it's also possible to get hurt while cleaning your garage, giving birth or driving a car. You can even choke while eating a kale salad. Does that mean we shouldn't do these things?

Despite what some say, I'm a true believer that the chances of getting injured if you work out are *much lower than if you don't work out.* Makes sense, right?

We are constantly subjected to fearmongering tactics perpetrated by the media, even (especially?) the fitness industry itself. That's right, my people: Most of the commercial fitness industry *does not actually want you to work out!* That's why there are pieces of equipment like abs machines, for example, that are built to isolate muscles that cannot be completely isolated. Or why treadmills are designed to give the *illusion* of exertion (fat burning zone?) but not to actually get you in shape.

It's also why gyms sign up new members every day but never get any more crowded week-to-week. They'd go out of business if all their members actually got results (or even showed up). Better to sign you up, tell you what you want to hear and send you on your way. Thank you, *DON'T* come again.

The real deal is that people respond to fear. When it snows, the news tells you to go out and stock up on groceries and shovels or you'll die an icy death. Conversely, when it's hot out—and a slow news day—similar threats are made about the perils of heat. For shame.

Ultimately, it's the individual's choice what to accept, inspiration or fear. The truth is that it's incredibly unlikely you will inflict bodily harm while training. A plane can crash, but flying is still the safest way to travel. I've even fallen off my bicycle, but I still ride it every day. It's still good for me.

Sure, a day (or even a week) off can be a good thing. But you don't necessarily have to plan for it or measure it with a slide rule. And you certainly don't need to be afraid to work out intensely or frequently. Let your body, life and experience dictate. Simply put, if your legs are aching, then train your arms. Your body gives you signals; listen to it. It's wiser than you think.

We all need to recover at times; I'd never deny it. As far as healing goes, respect your level. Though I sometimes *feel* like I have an adamantium skeleton, I don't. So when those moments arise when I need to back off, I do. No biggie. Common sense prevails yet again.

I've been practicing calisthenics for over 25 years and I've never suffered more than temporary discomfort (mostly from bumping my head on the pull-up bar or other such carelessness). Some tendonitis is the worst injury I've ever gotten, which is relatively minor on the grand scale.

And if we do get injured, no, we don't have supernatural healing powers, so pay attention to what you're experiencing. Embrace every moment with care. Be aware of what's around you. These practices are helpful in all aspects of life, not just fitness.

The Best Motivational Tip Ever

—By Al Kavadlo

Author's Insight—

There are essentially two types of fitness articles; the first gives advice on a specific exercise, program or protocol. These articles are great because they provide actionable ideas to improve specific aspects of our training. These are often some of my favorite articles.

The second doesn't really teach you anything about technique or exercise selection, but rather provides insight into the psychological forces behind our physical achievements. I tend to like these types of articles even better.

Danny and I were both personal trainers for a long time before we were ever fitness models, authors or presenters. And though we initially rose to prominence for our performance of a move known as the human flag, there was once a time when the flag seemed very much out of my reach.

This article explains the psychology behind how Danny and I have pushed each other towards new feats of strength over the years (like the flag), and how we continue to inspire those who we are fortunate enough to coach in person.

It's amazing what you can achieve with a little help from friends.

Before I ever performed a human flag, it seemed otherworldly and totally out of my reach. I'd seen the flag in photographs or videos, but I'd never actually seen it performed in real life, which only added to the mystique. That all changed the first time I saw my brother Danny Kavadlo perform the move in the flesh.

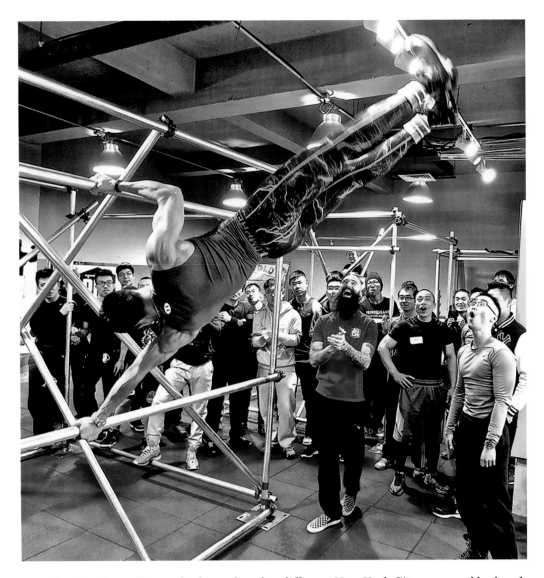

At the time, he and I were both employed at different New York City gyms and had each been practicing the flag on our own. After having recently discovered this amazing feat of strength online, we made an agreement with each other that we were both going to learn the human flag come hell or high water.

Since neither of us had access to a proper pole at our respective gyms, we were each trying to learn the human flag on the side posts of various workout machines. A few weeks had passed since we had committed ourselves toward this ambitious goal when Danny and I finally had our first opportunity to train together. Though I hadn't really gotten anywhere with the move yet on my own, Danny had clearly been attacking his human flag training with great tenacity. He grabbed the side of a cable machine with a look of determination and, to my amazement, pressed himself into a human flag.

Though Danny only managed to hold the position for a couple of seconds that day, it was long enough to ignite a fire deep inside of me. It was one thing to know that some faraway gymnast on the internet could do a human flag; it was quite another to see my own flesh and blood doing a human flag right before my eyes!

Once I saw Danny do the flag, it didn't take long for me to achieve the feat myself. I became more motivated to train than ever, since it no longer appeared to be out of reach. A similar thing happened the first time I saw a muscle-up: It provided tremendous motivation, and not very long after that, I achieved the move myself.

Danny and I now travel the globe teaching the human flag and other advanced calisthenics exercises to fitness trainers and enthusiasts, and we witness the same phenomenon at each and every workshop we instruct. Whether it's the flag, the handstand, the pistol squat or any of the other bodyweight skills we teach, there is always a steady stream of personal records set throughout the weekend.

I'm sure our students benefit from our helping them understand the proper technique for an exercise. That's huge. But I think the main reason so many people accomplish multiple PRs at our workshops has to do with something bigger than our experience or coaching ability.

You see, the number one factor that leads to these individual breakthroughs is the collective energy of the group. There is no form of motivation more powerful than simply seeing another human being do the very thing that you are trying to accomplish. Watching a "regular person" do something extraordinary has an uncanny way of suddenly demystifying it. Especially if that person is your friend, family member and/or training partner. Though professional athletes can appear superhuman at times, it's easy to look at someone you know in everyday life and say to yourself, "If they can do it, I can do it!"

If you are lacking motivation, I urge you to find others to inspire you. Whether it comes from attending a Progressive Calisthenics Certification, organizing a meet-up at your local park or hiring a personal trainer to help push you during your workouts, the motivation that comes from the presence of another human being will always trump that which can be provided by a mantra, video or article—even this one.

So what are you waiting for? Get off your butt, find some people to train with and get inspired!

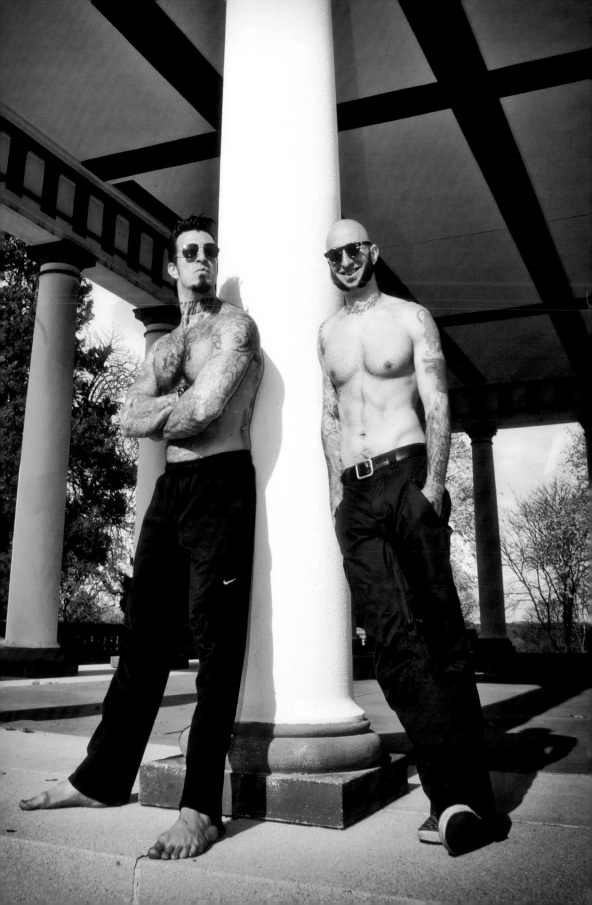

ABOUT THE AUTHORS

Al and Danny Kavadlo are two of the world's leading authorities on calisthenics and personal training. The Kavadlo Brothers have authored several internationally-acclaimed, bestselling books and have been translated into over a dozen languages. They have appeared in numerous publications including The New York Times and Men's Health, and are regular contributors to Bodybuilding.com and TRAIN magazine. As Master Instructors for Dragon Door's acclaimed Progressive Calisthenics Certification, Al and Danny travel the world teaching bodyweight strength training to athletes, professional trainers and fitness enthusiasts from all walks of life. They want you to *Get Strong*!

ALSO AVAILABLE FROM THE KAVADLO BROTHERS AND DRAGON DOOR:

Street Workout—A Worldwide Anthology of Urban Calisthenics—How to Sculpt a God-like Physique Using Nothing but Your Environment

By Al Kavadlo & Danny Kavadlo, 2016

Strength Rules—How to Get Stronger Than Almost Anyone and the Proven Plan to Make it Real

By Danny Kavadlo, 2015

Zen Mind, Strong Body—How to Cultivate Advanced Calisthenics Strength–Using the Power of "Beginner's Mind"

By Al Kavadlo, 2015

Diamond-Cut Abs—How to Engineer the Ultimate Six-Pack—Minimalist Methods for Maximal Results By Danny Kavadlo, 2014

Stretching Your Boundaries—Flexibility Training for Extreme Calisthenic Strength

By Al Kavadlo, 2014

Everybody Needs Training—Proven Success Secrets for Fitness Professionals—How to Get More Clients, Make More Money and Change More Lives

By Danny Kavadlo, 2013

Pushing The Limits!—Total Body Strength with No Equipment

By Al Kavadlo, 2013

Raising The Bar—The Definitive Guide to Pull-up Bar Calisthenics

By Al Kavadlo, 2012

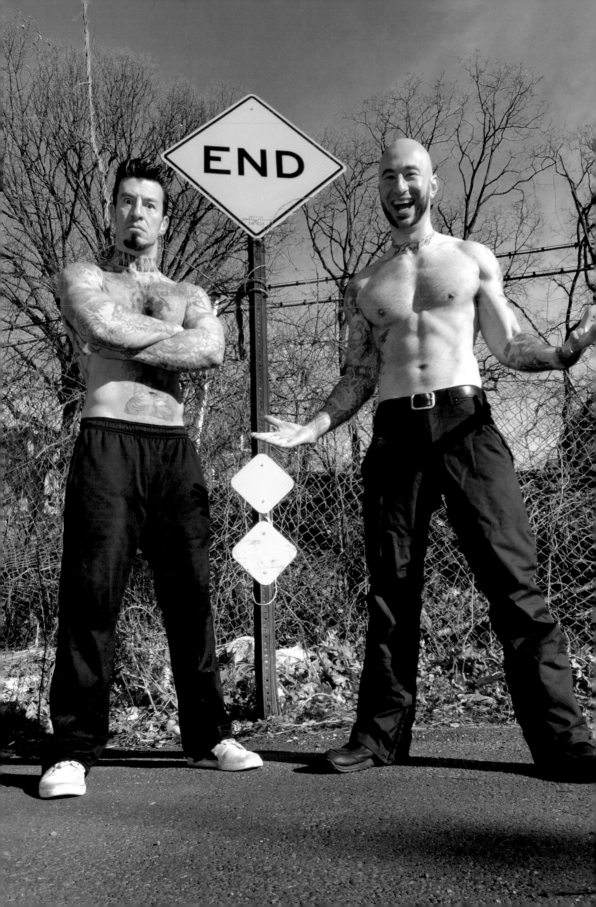

INDEX OF EXERCISES

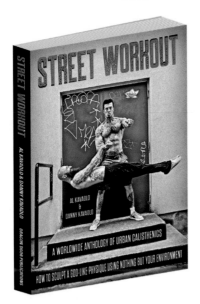

STREET WORKOUT
A WORLDWIDE ANTHOLOGY
OF URBAN CALISTHENICS

Street Workout
A Worldwide Anthology
of Urban Calisthenics:
How to Sculpt a God-Like
Physique Using Nothing
But Your Environment
By Al Kavadlo and
Danny Kavadlo

Book #B87 $34.95
eBook #EB87 $19.95
Paperback 6.75 x 9.5
406 pages, 305 photos

"Al and Danny Kavadlo—bodyweight coaches extraordinaire—have done it again. Their new book *Street Workout* is an incredibly comprehensive collection of calisthenics concepts, exercises and programs. In addition to their masterful demonstrations of every exercise, the Kavadlo brothers' colorful personalities and motivational talents leap off of every page. If you're serious about bodyweight training, you've gotta get this book!"**—MARK SISSON**, author of *The Primal Blueprint*

"Al and Danny Kavadlo are acknowledged worldwide as masters of urban bodyweight training, so it's no surprise that this book is, without question, the new "bible" of the movement. This work is the greatest manual on progressive calisthenics available on the market today. It's loaded with incredible progressions, stacked with tips and techniques, and overflowing with philosophy and wisdom. The programming sections are beyond extensive. *Street Workout* is THE magnum opus of the two greatest calisthenics coaches on the planet today. All serious athletes and coaches must buy this book!!"**—PAUL "COACH" WADE**, author of *Convict Conditioning*

"I truly LOVE this book—it is utterly sensational and brilliant! Al and Danny Kavadlo have a fun and informative way of explaining and demonstrating the key calisthenics exercises for a fit, healthy and happy life. Their sharp instructional images are joyfully inspirational and always motivate me to bust out some reps on the spot! I truly wish there had been a comprehensive workout guide like this when I first discovered the miracles of bodyweight training."**—MARCUS BONDI**, two time Official Guinness World Record Holder (weighted chin-ups & rope climb)

"Once again, an outstanding addition to our field of fitness from Danny and Al. I am a barbell/kettlebell guy first and foremost, but the Kavadlo brothers have finally convinced me of the pure value of using the body only as load."**—DAN JOHN**, author of *Never Let Go*

"This book brings together the vast knowledge and experience of two guys that definitely embody the whole street workout culture—hardcore, sometimes gritty but always extremely welcoming, with a whole lot of individual style and flare."**—MIKE FITCH**, creator of *Global Bodyweight Training* and The *Animal Flow Workout*

Your Ultimate Guide to Full Body Fitness Without Weights: The Secrets of "Street Workout" Revealed…

How to Release Yourself from the Gym, Restore Your Primal Power and Reclaim Your Inner Beast…

According to the **Kavadlos**, working out should be fun, adventurous, primal and pure. And no training style embodies those elements quite like Street Workout. The outside world becomes your total gym—you roam free to get stronger using simply your own body and the environment at hand…

The great masters of *Street Workout* perform stunning physical feats that can intimidate lesser mortals. But the beauty of the Kavadlos' approach in *Street Workout* is to make even the toughest moves achievable by any enthusiast willing to follow their guidelines. *Street Workout's* multi-faceted, progressive approach leaves nothing to chance— allowing even a raw beginner to transcend his mortal frame and ascend to the giddiest heights of physical supremacy…

Intermediate and advanced calisthenics practitioners will discover a veritable treasure chest of tips, techniques and insider secrets—guaranteed to force-feed their future achievements in the realm of bodyweight mastery.

Pushing, pulling and squatting your own bodyweight along with forward flexion and back bridging represent the basics of getting brutally strong, solid and unbreakable. By utilizing basic principles of progression such as the manipulation of leverage, adding or removing points of contact and/or increasing the range of motion, you can continue to get stronger without ever having to pick up a weight—and have a helluva good time while you're at it!

Street Workout proves it so—with its mix of inspirational photography, exact detail on what to do when—and its step-by-step blueprints for off-the-charts, eye-popping physical excellence.

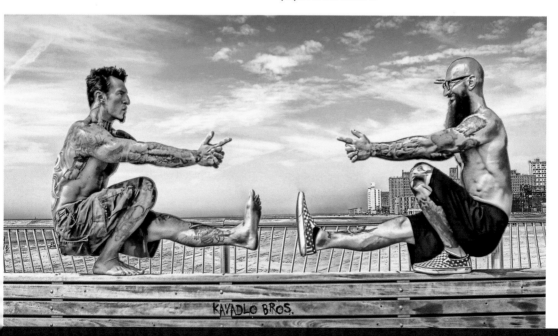

KAVADLO BROS.

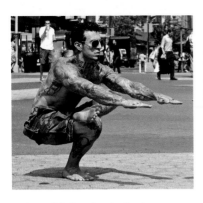
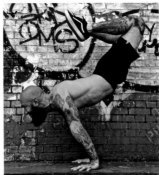
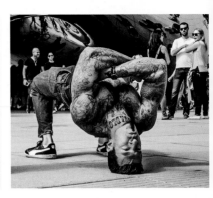

Street Workout fires its first barrage with a crucial section on the **Foundational Progressions**—future and ongoing physical greatness cannot be achieved without mastery of these five fundamental pillars of fitness…

You will immediately appreciate the nobility, virtue and integrity of these movement patterns. Absorb the wisdom of this first section and you have absorbed the very heart and soul of the Street Workout ethos…

CHAPTER 4 awards you the foundational progressions for the **Push**—in all its glory. Discover 30 different progressive drills from the Plank to the Claw Push-Up, to the One-Arm Push-Up to the Hindu Press, to the Ultimate Headstand Press to the Bench Dip to the Korean Dip…

Master all of these 30 moves and you can already tag yourself as a Monster :)

CHAPTER 5 awards you the foundational progressions for the **Pull**—and we're all here for the Pull-Up right? Discover 26 different progressive drills from the Bent-Knee Aussie to the Flex Hang, to the Commando Pull-Up, to the L Pull-Up, to the One-Arm Pull Up…

Look, there is no substitute in strength training for the pull-up—all the more so in our hunched-over world of addiction to devices… And mastery of Chapter 5 earns you the Maestro tag for sure…

CHAPTER 6 awards you the foundational progressions for the Squat—the ultimate movement needed to build jack hammer legs. Discover 28 different progressive drills from the Bench-Assisted Squat, to the Prisoner Squat, to the Archer Squat, to the Drinking Bird, to the Pole-Assisted Pistol to the Dragon Pistol, to the Advanced Shrimp to the Hawaiian Squat…

Let's face it, you are not a real man or woman without a powerful pair of posts—you are more of a liability to the species… Master this section and you get to represent the species with the Superman or Superwoman tag…

CHAPTER 7 awards you the foundational progressions for the **Flex**—meaning "full body forward flexion". Discover 19 different progressive drills from the Lying Knee Tuck, to the L-Sit, to the Dragon Flag, to the Hanging Leg Raise, to the Rollover, to the Meathook…

Master this section and your etched abs and ripped upper-body musculature will earn you the Mister or Madam Magnificent tag… :)

CHAPTER 8 awards you the foundational progressions for the **Bridge**. Discover 15 different progressive drills from the Hip Bridge, to the Candlestick Straight Bridge, to the One Leg Back Bridge, to the Stand-to-Stand Bridge…

Bridging is an invaluable yet often overlooked component of full body fitness. Bridge work will have a dramatic impact on your power, balance and flexibility—and give you a back that would make a wild tiger proud…

Master this section—along with the previous four—and you can consider your Manhood or Womanhood beyond serious challenge…

So—thanks to mastering the five foundational keys of full body fitness—you can now count yourself as more magnificently in shape than 99% of the human race. But Street Workout encourages you to not stop there, not rest on your laurels…

If you've got this far, then why not shoot for the stars—and enter the immortal ranks of the top 1% of the planet's physical specimens? You can do it! As **Al Kavadlo** and **Danny Kavadlo** themselves bear witness—in photo after photo after photo…

Time to introduce the **SKILLS & "TRICKS"** section of *Street Workout*…

Mastering the exercise progressions in this section will propel you to new heights, to the land where the giants of *Street Workout* strut their splendid stuff. And make no mistake, only the bold of heart, the iron-willed and the profoundly persistent will be godlike enough to make it all the way… If you have those qualities, then nothing should stop you—because the complete blueprint for mastery is laid out for you…

If you are one of those folk looking for cheap hacks so you can pretend your way to greater strength, then this section of *Street Workout* is not for you… However, if you are made of sterner stuff, then read on…

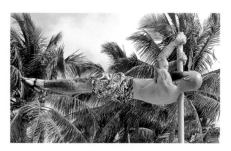 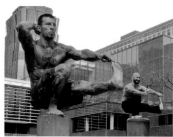 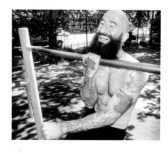

Exercises like the muscle-up, the handstand or the human flag demand the perfect mix of technical skill, hard training and thousands of progressive reps to attain. The Floor Holds, Bar Moves and Human Flag categories within this section contain the instructions you need to make it to the summit. The rest is up to you…

CHAPTER 9 awards you the progressions for Floor Holds. Discover 34 different progressive drills from the Frog Stand, to the One Arm/One Leg Crow, to the Ultimate Headstand, to the Straddle Handstand, to the One Arm handstand, to the One Arm Elbow Lever, to the Scorpion Planche…

The final category to achieve here is the Planche which represents calisthenics strength, precision, skill and fortitude in the most advanced forms. Have at it and let us know how you do!

CHAPTER 10 awards you the progressions for Bar Moves. Discover 20 different progressive drills from the Muscle-Up, to Skinning the Cat, to the Back Lever, to the Front Lever…

Nothing screams *"Street Workout"* like bar moves. Many practitioners of advanced calisthenics were roped in the first time they saw these exercises because they are so spectacular looking. The Kavadlos sure were!

However, these bar moves are not just eye-poppingly cool to look at—they require tremendous strength, skill and perseverance to attain. These gravity-defying feats will suspend you in mid-air and have you feeling like king or queen of the world!

CHAPTER 11 awards you the progressions for the **Human Flag**. Discover 25 different progressive drills from the Side Plank, to the Clutch Flag, to the Support Press, to the Vertical Flag, to the Human Flag Crucifix, to the One Arm Flag, to the Human Flag…

The full press flag has become synonymous with Street Workout. Perform it in public and watch as heads swivel, jaws drop, hearts pound and iPhones leap into action like there's no tomorrow!

Again, though, beyond the amazing visual, there is an ungodly amount of upper body strength needed to perform the numerous types of human flag. Flags will give you—and require—beastly arms, shoulders, an iron chest and a back of sprung steel. The good news is that this chapter lays out the complete blueprint on how to go from Flag-newbie to Human Flag hellraiser…

SECTION IV of *Street Workout* addresses the crucial matter of Programming…

CHAPTER 12 gives you a handy set of **Assessments** so you can see how you stack up against the best in the bodyweight kingdom. Here you can assess your relative calisthenics competency across a broad array of classic street workout exercises. These charts can also serve as a guideline to help you determine when it is appropriate to move on to harder exercises.

CHAPTER 13, Street Workouts, gives you

12 routines to follow or adapt that run from moderate to diabolical in their intensity…

Go from the modest **Start Me Up**, take the **50 Rep Challenge**, say hello to the **Three Amigos,** charge yourself up with **Static Electricity**, split yourself in half with **Up Above** and **Down Below**, bring it and bear it with the Full Frontal, be a sucker for punishment with **Back For More**, magically get the highest possible strength gains with the **Wizard's Cauldron**, scorch your upper body with **Danny's Inferno**, brutalize your horrified posts with **Leg Daze** and finally—for the ultimate of Street Workout warrior challenges—take on the **Destroyer of Worlds!**

CHAPTER 14 gives you 6 **Training Templates** that you can incorporate into your programming. They serve as examples of how you can approach your routines.

A final **BONUS SECTION** brings invaluable additional advice from Al and Danny which pulls the whole Street Workout shebang together, based on questions they've been asked over the years as trainers.

Street Workout
A Worldwide Anthology of Urban Calisthenics: How to Sculpt a God-Like Physique Using Nothing But Your Environment
By Al Kavadlo and Danny Kavadlo

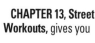

Book #B87 $34.95
eBook #EB87 $19.95
Paperback 6.75 x 9.5
406 pages, 305 photos

How to Get Stronger Than Almost Anyone— And The Proven Plan to Make It Real

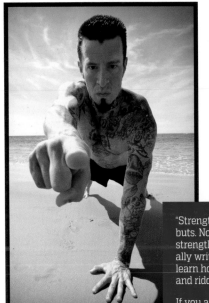

"Strength Rules is one of the finest books on strength I've ever read. No ifs, ands or buts. Not just 'bodyweight strength'—*strength*, period. There are a million and one strength books out there about hoisting heavy iron and screwing up your joints...usually written by coaches and athletes using steroids and other drugs. But if you want to learn how to unleash *ferocious* strength and power while also improving your health and ridding yourself of extra fat and joint pain, THIS is the book you need to own.

If you are a bodyweight master, this is the bible you will want to go back to again and again, to keep you on the straight and narrow. If you are raw beginner—Jeez, then get this book right now, *follow the rules*, and save yourself years of wasted effort! Strength Rules is as good as it gets!"
—**PAUL WADE**, author of *Convict Conditioning*

How to Be Tough as Nails— Whatever You Do, Wherever You Go, Whenever You Need it...

Want to get *classically* strong—in every dimension of your life— gut, heart and mind...?

In other words, do you want to be:
- **More than** just gym-strong?
- **More than** just functionally strong?
- **More than** just sport-specifically strong?
- **More than** just butt-kicker strong?
- And—certainly—**more than** just look-pretty-in-a-bodybuilding-contest strong?

Do you demand—instead—to be:
- **Tensile Strong?**
- **Versatile Strong?**
- **Pound-for-Pound Strong?**
- **The Ultimate Physical Dynamo?**
- **A Mental Powerhouse?**
- **A Spiritual Force?**
- **An Emotional Rock?**

Then welcome to **Danny's World**... the world of *Strength Rules*— where you can stand tall on a rock-solid foundation of classic strength principles...Arm-in-arm with a world leader in the modern calisthenics movement...

Then... with Danny as your constant guide, grow taller and ever-stronger—in all aspects of your life and being—with a Master Blueprint of progressive calisthenic training where the sky's the limit on your possible progress...

Do Danny's classical **Strength Rules**—and, for sure, you can own the keys to the strength kingdom...

Ignore Danny's classical **Strength Rules**—break them, twist them, lame-ass them, screw with them—then doom yourself to staying stuck in idle as a perpetual strength mediocrity...

The choice is yours!

"I have been waiting for a book to be written on strength training that I can recommend to all of my patients, and **Danny Kavadlo** has delivered with **Strength Rules**. Danny has written a stripped down approach to strength that is accessible to everyone.

He has distilled his wealth of knowledge and experience in coaching and bodyweight strength training into a program that is cohesive, scalable, and instantly applicable to all comers. He has also added a rock solid approach to nutrition and ample doses of inspirational story telling and philosophy, resulting in the gem that is **Strength Rules**.

I dare anyone to read this book and still give me an excuse why they can't strengthen their body and improve their health. No excuses. Get the book and get to work!"
—**DR. CHRISTOPHER HARDY**, author of *Strong Medicine*

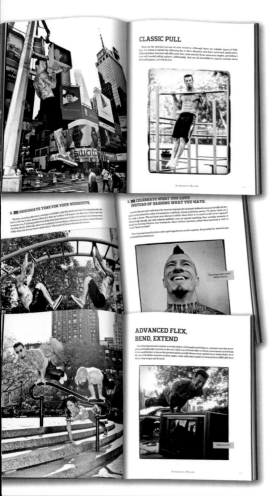

However brilliant most strength books might be, 99% of them have a fatal flaw...

99% of otherwise excellent strength books focus on only one aspect of strength: how to get physically stronger through physical exercise. Health and multi-dimensional well-being is given at best a cursory nod... Nutritional advice is most often a thinly disguised pitch for a supplement line...

If you want a book that gives you the goods on full-body training, full-body health and full-body strength, then there's precious little out there... So, thank God for the advent of *Strength Rules*!

Strength Rules embodies all elements of strength—even how they work into our day-to-day existence, the highs and lows of our being, for better or for worse...

Strength Rules is dedicated to those who are down with the cause. Those who want to work hard to get strong. Who insist they deserve to build their own muscle, release their own endorphins and synthesize *their own* hormones.

Strength Rules has no interest in fly-by-night fitness fads. Classic exercises have stood the test of time for a reason. *Strength Rules* shouts a loud "just say no!" to cumbersome, complicated workout equipment. *Strength Rules* walks a path free from trendy diets, gratuitous chemical concoctions and useless gear...

Almost every strength exercise comes down to the basics. Essentially, Squat, Push and Pull. These three broad, essential movements are the granddaddies of 'em all. Throw in some Flexion, Transverse Bends and Extension, and you've got yourself the tools for a lifetime of full body strength training... That's why the exercises contained in *Strength Rules* are divided into these few, broad categories. Everything else is a variation. There is no reason to overcomplicate it.

The *Strength Rules* mission is to help anybody and everybody get in the best shape of their lives Strength Rules lays out the truth clearly and succinctly, giving you the tools you need to grow stronger and persevere in this mad world—with your head held high and your body lean and powerful...

The exercise portion of *Strength Rules* (titled ACTIONS) is split into three levels: Basic Training (Starting Out), Beast Mode (Classic Strength) and Like A Boss (Advanced Moves). Naturally, not everyone will fall 100% into one of these groups for all exercises in all categories and that's fine. In fact, it's likely that even the same individual's level will vary from move to move. That's cool; we all progress at different rates. Respect and acknowledge it. Trust your instincts.

Speaking of instincts, we are wired with them for a reason. If our instincts are wrong then that's millions of years of evolution lying to us. A large part of *Strength Rules* embraces empowerment, faith in oneself and emotional awareness. Danny believes that being honest with yourself, physically, mentally and spiritually is a magnificent (and necessary) component of true, overall strength. Yes, sometimes the truth hurts, but it must be embraced if we are ever to be fit and free. We all have the power within ourselves. Use it.

Strength Rules cries out to all body types, age groups, backgrounds and disciplines. It talks to the beginning student. It calls on the advanced practitioner, looking for new challenges. It speaks to the calisthenics enthusiast and all the hard-working personal trainers... *Strength Rules* is for *everyone* who wants to get strong—and then some...

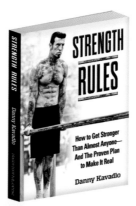

Strength Rules
How to Get Stronger Than Almost Anyone— And The Proven Plan to Make It Real
By Danny Kavadlo

Book #B84 $39.99
eBook #EB84 $9.99
Paperback 8.5 x 11
264 pages, 305 photos

Most folk who embark on a career as a trainer, do so initially out of a personal passion for fitness and a strong desire to help other achieve results. Be it weight loss, conditioning, strength gains, flexibility or enhanced performance.

But a passion for working out and an earnest desire to help others—alone—does not a successful personal trainer make. The sad fact is that the turn over rate for personal trainers after one year is over 80%. Why? It's almost always because the trainer didn't have a proper understanding of the BUSINESS of being a fitness professional.

The bottom line is that without the appropriate success blueprint, the most skilled and knowledgeable personal trainer is usually doomed to failure. Unfortunately, until now, there has been no such battle-tested blueprint available either to the novice trainer or the professional struggling to stay alive. Now, however that's all changed, thanks to Danny Kavadlo's *Everybody Needs*

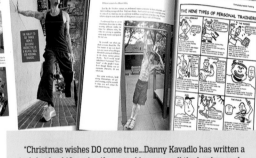

"*Everybody Needs Training* is quite 'something.' I don't think I have ever seen this kind of depth in the field. It's both obvious and 'wow' as you read it. Amazing stuff. It fills a gap in the community that, frankly, surprises me no one has really filled."—**DAN JOHN**, author, *Never Let Go*

"Danny Kavadlo has personally helped me become a more successful trainer and coach. I cannot recommend *Everybody Needs Training* enough. It's the best book I've ever seen on the subject of being a professional trainer." —**ADEL GABER**, World Class Trainer & 3-Time Olympic Wrestling Coach

"*Everybody Needs Training* is a solid collection of tried-and-true best practices that can help personal trainers on any level reach their full potential in their chosen field."—**ROLANDO GARCIA**, RKC II, CK-FMS

"*Everybody Needs Training* is a must-read for every personal trainer wanting to take it to the next level, and everyone who has ever dreamed of becoming a personal trainer. This book allows you to get inside the genius PT mind of Danny Kavadlo, a master of his craft, speaking off the cuff to you about training—priceless!"—**ERRICK MCADAMS**, Personal Trainer, Model, Fitness Personality

"Christmas wishes DO come true....Danny Kavadlo has written a training book! Imagine if you could squeeze all the hard-earned wisdom, secrets and tactics of one of the world's hottest personal trainers between the covers of a beautifully illustrated tell-all manual, and you have imagined *Everybody Needs Training*.

Like Danny himself, this groundbreaking book is incredibly smart, brutally honest, laugh-out-loud funny, and totally out of left field...if you train others (casually or professionally), want a career training others, or if you just love the now-famous "Kavadlo approach" to getting in shape, you owe it to yourself to grab a copy of this masterpiece. I cannot recommend it highly enough." —**PAUL WADE**, author of *Convict Conditioning*

Good for any profession or business

"I'm not a trainer, but took Danny and Al's PCC Class. This is a great book for anyone going into business as either an employee or owner, whether a fitness trainer or any other kind of business. I'm a lawyer, and I'm thinking about making it required reading for my newly hired lawyers. Good practical advice, with the focus on the customer, which is a focus that seems to be lost these days. Easy reading, but pithy, with lots of great tips and ideas, with an excellent overriding theme. Oh yea -- well written too!"—**Mark Walker,** McAllen, Texas

Everybody Needs Training
Proven Success Secrets for the Professional Fitness Trainer—How to Get More Clients, Make More Money, Change More Lives
By Danny Kavadlo

Book #B72 $34.95
eBook #EB72 $19.95
Paperback 8.5 x 11

C-MASS

How To Maximize Muscle Growth Using Bodyweight-Only

I s it really possible to add significant extra muscle-bulk to your frame using bodyweight exercise only? The answer, according to calisthenics guru and bestselling *Convict Conditioning* author Paul Wade, is a resounding Yes. Legendary strongmen and savvy modern bodyweight bodybuilders both, have added stacks of righteous beef to their physiques—using just the secrets Paul Wade reveals in this bible-like guide to getting as strong AND as big as you could possibly want, using nothing but your own body.

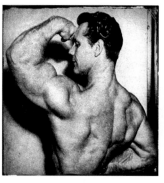 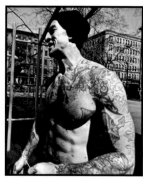

Paul Wade's trenchant, visceral style blazes with hard-won body culture insight, tactics, strategies and tips for the ultimate blueprint for getting huge naturally without free weights, machine supplements or—God forbid—steroids. With *C-Mass*, Paul Wade further cements his position as the preeminent modern authority on how to build extraordinary power and strength with bodyweight exercise only.

⬇ Get All of This When You Invest in Paul Wade's *C-Mass* Today: ⬇

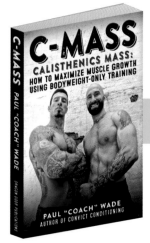

C-MASS
Calisthenics Mass: How To Maximize Muscle Growth Using Bodyweight-Only Training
By Paul "Coach" Wade

Book #B75 $24.95

eBook #EB75 $9.95

Paperback 8.5 x 11 • 136 pages, 130 photos

1. Bodyweight Muscle? No Problem!

Build *phenomenal* amounts of natural muscle mass and discover how to:

- Add 20-30+ pounds of solid muscle—with perfect proportions
- Reshape your arms with 2-3 inches of gnarly beef
- Triple the size of your pecs and lats
- Thicken and harden your abdominal wall into a classic six-pack
- Throw a thick, healthy vein onto your biceps
- Generate hard, sculpted quads and hamstrings that would be the envy of an Olympic sprinter
- Build true "diamond" calves
- Stand head and shoulders above the next 99% of natural bodybuilders in looks, strength and power
- Boost your testosterone naturally to bull-like levels

Understand the radically different advantages you'll get from the two major types of resistance work, *nervous system* training and *muscular system* training.

If you really want to explode your muscle growth—if SIZE is your goal—you should train THIS way...

2. The Ten Commandments of Calisthenics Mass

Truly effective muscular training boils down into THESE Ten Commandments.

COMMANDMENT I: Embrace reps!

Why reps are key when you want to build massive stacks of jacked up muscle.

Understanding the biochemistry of building bigger muscles through reps...

COMMANDMENT II: Work Hard!

Want to turn from a twig into an ok tree? Why working demonically hard and employing brutal physical effort is essential to getting nasty big...

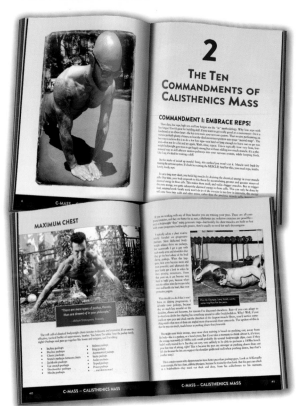

MAXIMUM CHEST

COMMANDMENT III:
Use Simple, Compound Exercises!

Why—if you want to get swole—you need to toss out complex, high-skill exercises.

Why *dynamic* exercises are generally far better than *static holds* for massive muscle building.

These are the very best dynamic exercises—for bigger bang for your muscle buck.

How to ratchet up the heat with THIS kick-ass strategy and sprout new muscle at an eye-popping rate.

COMMANDMENT IV:
Limit Sets!

What it takes to trigger explosive muscle growth—and why most folk foolishly and wastefully pull their "survival trigger" way too many futile times...

Why you need to void "volume creep" at all costs when size is what you're all about.

COMMANDMENT V: Focus on Progress—and Utilize a Training Journal!

Why so few wannabe athletes ever achieve a good level of strength and muscle—let alone a *great* level—and what it really takes to succeed.

Golden tip: how to take advantage of the *windows of opportunity* your training presents you.

How to transform miniscule, incremental gains into long-range massive outcomes.

Forgot those expensive supplements! Why keeping a training log can be the missing key to success or failure in the muscle-gain biz.

COMMANDMENT VI: You Grow When You Rest. So Rest!

If you *really* wanted to improve on your last workout—add that rep, tighten up your form—how would you want to approach that workout? The answer is right here...

Ignore THIS simple, ancient, muscle-building fact—and be prepared to go on spinning your muscle-building wheels for a VERY long time...

10 secrets to optimizing the magic rest-muscle growth formula...

Why you may never even come close to your full physical potential—but how to change that...

COMMANDMENT VII: Quit Eating "Clean" the Whole Time!

Warning—Politically incorrect statement: Why, if you are trying to pack on more muscle, eating junk now and again is not only okay, it can be positively *anabolic*.

COMMANDMENT VIII:
Sleep More!

How is it that prison athletes seem to gain and maintain so much dense muscle, when guys on the outside—who are taking supplements and working out in super-equipped gyms—can rarely gain muscle at all?

Discover the 3 main reasons why, sleep, the natural alternative to steroids, helps prison athletes grow so big...

COMMANDMENT IX: Train the Mind Along With the Body!

Why your mind is your most powerful supplement...

How 6 major training demons can destroy your bodybuilding dreams—and where to find the antidote...

COMMANDMENT X:
Get Strong!

Understanding the relationship between the nervous system and the muscular system—and how to take full advantage of that relationship.

Why, if you wish to gain as much muscle as your genetic potential will allow, just training your *muscles* won't cut it—and what more you need to do...

The secret to mixing and matching for both growth AND strength...

3. "Coach" Wade's Bodypart Tactics

Get the best bodyweight bodybuilding techniques for 11 major body areas.

1. Quadzilla! (...and Quadzookie.)

Why the Gold Standard quad developer is squatting—and why you absolutely need to master the Big Daddy, the *one-legged squat*...

How to perform the Shrimp Squat, a wonderful quad and glute builder, which is comparable to the one-leg squat in terms of body-challenge.

Why you should employ THESE 7 jumping methods to put your quad gains through the roof...

How to perform the hyper-tough, man-making Sissy Squat—favorite of the Iron Guru, Vince Gironda—great bodybuilding ideologist of the Golden Era, and trainer of a young Mr. Schwarzenegger. He wouldn't let anyone perform barbell squats in his gym!

2. Hamstrings: Stand Sideways With Pride

Enter *Lombard's Paradox*: how and why you can successfully brutalize your hammies with calisthenics.

Why bridging is a perfect exercise for strengthening the hamstrings.

How to correctly work your hamstrings and activate your entire posterior chain.

Why THIS workout of straight bridges and hill sprints could put muscle on a pencil.

How to employ the little-known secret of the *bridge curl* to develop awesome strength and power in the your hammies.

Why explosive work is essential for fully developed hamstrings—and the best explosive exercise to make your own...

3. Softball Biceps

THIS is the best biceps exercise in the world, *bar none*. But most bodybuilders never use it to build their biceps! Discover what you are missing out on and learn to do it right...

And then you can make dumbbell curls look like a redheaded stepchild with THIS superior bicep blower-upper...

Another great compound move for the biceps (and forearms) is *rope climbing*. As with all bodyweight, this can be performed progressively. Get the details here on why and how...

Despite what some trainers may ignorantly tell you, you can also perform bodyweight biceps *isolation* exercises—such as the classic (but-rarely-seen-in-gyms) *curl-up*. Pure power! If you can build one, THIS old school piece of kit will give you biceps straight from Hades.

4. Titanic Triceps

Paul Wade has *never* met a gym-trained bodybuilder who understands how the triceps work. Not one. Learn how the triceps REALLY work. This stuff is gold—pay attention. And discover the drills that are going to CRUCIFY those tris!

4. Farmer Forearms

Paul Wade wrote the definitive mini-manual of calisthenics forearm and grip training in *Convict Conditioning 2*. But HERE'S a reminder on the take-home message that forearms are best built through THESE exercises, and you can build superhuman grip utilizing intelligent THESE progressions...

Why crush-style grippers are a mistake and the better, safer alternative for a hand-punishing grip...

5. It's Not "Abs", It's "Midsection"

As a bodybuilder, your method should be to pick a big, tough midsection movement and work at it hard and progressively to thicken your six-pack. This work should be a cornerstone of your training, no different from pullups or squats. It's a requirement! Which movements to pick? Discover the drills here...

And the single greatest exercise for scorching your abs in the most effective manner possible is THIS...

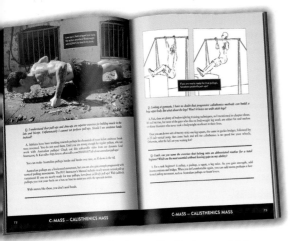

How to best train your obliques and lateral chain...

The simplest and most effective way to train your transversus...

6. Maximum Chest

The roll call of classical bodyweight chest exercises is dynamic and impressive. It's an ancient, effective, tactical buffet of super-moves. Get the list here...

THE best chest routine is THIS one...

If super-sturdy arms and shoulders mean your pecs barely get a look in when you press, then focus on THESE progressions instead—and your pecs will be burning with a welcome new pain...

Why Al Kavadlo has a lean, athletic physique, but his pecs are as thick as a bodybuilder's...

THIS could be the ultimate bodyweight drill to get thick, imposing pectoral muscles...

And here's the single finest exercise for enlarging your pec minor—yet hardly anyone has figured it out...

Why you need to master the art of deep breathing, strongman style, to truly develop a massive chest—and where to find unbeatable advice from proven champions...

7. Powerful, Healthy Shoulders

All die-hard bodybuilders need to know is that the deltoids have three heads. Here's how they work...

If you want to give any of your shoulder heads an enhanced, specialist workout, a great tactic is THIS.

How to make your lateral deltoids scream for mercy—and thank you later when you ignore their pleas...

If you really want to build your rear delts, THIS drill should be your number one exercise...

THESE kinds of drills can result in shoulder injury, rotator cuff tears, frozen shoulder and chronic pain—what to stick with instead...

THIS is a fantastic deltoid movement which

will swell up those cannonballs fast...

Why old school hand balancing is so great for strength, size and coordination, while surprisingly easy on the shoulders, especially as you get a bit older...

The number one go-to guy in the whole world for hand-balancing is THIS calisthenics master...

8. Ah'll be Back

THIS exercise is the finest lat-widener in the bodybuilding world and should be the absolute mainstay of your back training. This one's a no-brainer—if adding maximum torso beef as fast and efficiently as possible appeals to you...

Are you an advanced bodyweight bodybuilder? Then you may wish to add THIS to your upper-back routine. Why? Well—THIS will blitz your rear delts, scapular muscles and the lower heads of the trapezius. These are the "detail" muscles of the back, so loved by bodybuilders when they grow and thicken, resembling serpents swirling around the shoulder-blades.

Paul Wade demands that all his students begin their personal training with a brutal regime of THIS punishing drill. Why? Find out here...

Real strength monsters can try THIS. But you gotta be real powerful to survive the attempt...

Many bodybuilders think only in terms of "low back" when working the spinal muscles, but this is a mistake: find out why...

How bridging fully works all the deep tissues of the spine and bulletproofs the discs.

The single most effective bridge technique for building massive back muscle...

Why back levers performed THIS way are particularly effective in building huge spinal strength and thickness.

Why inverse hyperextensions are a superb lower-back and spine exercise which requires zero equipment.

9. Calving Season

THIS squat method will make your calves larger, way more supple, more powerful, and your ankles/Achilles' tendon will be bulletproofed like a steel cable...

Whether you are an athlete, a strength trainer or a pure bodyweight bodybuilder, your first mission should be to gradually build to THIS. Until you get there, you don't need to waste time on any specialist calf exercises.

If you DO want to add specific calf exercises to your program, then THESE are a good choice.

The calves are naturally explosive muscles, and explosive bodyweight work is very good for calf-building. So add THESE six explosive drills into your mix...

Methods like THIS are so brutal (and effective) that they can put an inch or more on stubborn calves in just weeks. If you can train like this just once a week for a few months, you better get ready to outgrow your socks...

10. TNT: Total Neck and Traps

Do bodybuilders even need to do neck work? Here's the answer...

The best neck exercises for beginners.

HERE is an elite-level technique for developing the upper trapezius muscles between the neck and shoulders..

THIS is another wonderful exercise for the traps, developing them from all angles.

By the time you can perform two sets of twenty deep, slow reps of THIS move, your traps will look like hardcore cans of beans.

If you want more neck, and filling out your collar is something you want to explore, forget those decapitation machines in the gym, or those headache-inducing head straps. The safest, most natural and most productive techniques for building a bull-nape are THESE.

4. Okay. Now Gimme a Program

If you want to pack on muscle using bodyweight, it's no good training like a gymnast or a martial artist or a dancer or a yoga expert, no matter how impressive those skill-based practitioners might be at performing advanced calisthenics. You need a different mindset. You need to train like a bodybuilder!

Learn the essential C-Mass principles behind programming, so you can master your own programming...

The most important thing to understand about bodybuilding routines...

Simple programs with minimum complexity have THESE features

By contrast, programs with maximum complexity have THESE features

Why Simple Beats Complex, For THESE 3 Very Important Reasons...

When to Move up the Programming Line

If simpler, more basic routines are always the best, why do advanced bodybuilders tend to follow more complex routines? Programs with different sessions for different bodyparts, with dozens of exercises? Several points to consider...

The best reason is to move up the programming line is THIS

Fundamental Program Templates

• Total Body 1, Total Body 2
• Upper/Lower-Body Split 1, Upper/Lower-Body Split 2
• 3-Way Split 1, 3-Way Split 2
• 4-Way Split 1, 4-Way Split 1

5. Troubleshooting Muscle-Growth: The FAQ

Q. Why bodyweight? Why can't I use weights and machines to build muscle?

Q. I understand that pull-ups and chin-ups are superior exercises for building muscle in the lats and biceps. Unfortunately I cannot yet perform pull-ups. Should I use assistance bands instead?

Q. Looking at gymnasts, I have no doubt that progressive calisthenics methods can build a huge upper body. But what about the legs? Won't it leave me with stick legs?

Q. Coach, can you name the exercises that belong into an abbreviated routine for a total beginner? Which are the most essential without leaving gaps in my ability?

Q. "Big" bodyweight exercises such as push-ups and pull-ups may target the larger muscles of the body (pecs, lats, biceps, etc.), but what about the smaller muscles which are still so important to the bodybuilder? Things like forearms, the calves, the neck?

Q. I have been told I need to use a weighted vest on my push-ups and pull-ups if I want to get stronger and gain muscle. Is this true?

Q. Is bodyweight training suitable for women? Do you know of any women who achieved the "Master Steps" laid out in Convict Conditioning?

Q. I am very interested in gaining size—not just muscle mass, but also height. Is it possible that calisthenics can increase my height?

Q. You have said that moving exercises are superior to isometrics when it comes to mass gain. I am interested in getting huge shoulders, but Convict Conditioning gives several static (isometric) exercises early on in the handstand pushup chain. Can you give me any moving exercises I can use instead, to work up to handstand pushups?

Q. *I have heard that the teenage years are the ideal age for building muscle. Is there any point in trying to build muscle after the age of forty?*

Q. *I have had some knee problems in the past; any tips for keeping my knee joints healthy so I can build more leg mass?*

Q. *I'm pretty skinny and I have always had a huge amount of trouble putting on weight—any weight, even fat. Building muscle is virtually impossible for me. What program should I be on?*

Q. *I've read in several bodybuilding magazines that I need to change my exercises frequently in order to "confuse" my muscles into growth. Is that true?*

Q. *I read in several bodybuilding magazines that I need to eat protein every 2-3 hours to have a hope in hell of growing. They also say that I need a huge amount of protein, like two grams per pound of bodyweight. Why don't your Commandments mention the need for protein?*

Q. *I have heard that whey is the "perfect" food for building muscle. Is this true?*

6. The Democratic Alternative…how to get as powerful as possible without gaining a pound

There is a whole bunch of folks who either want (or need) massive strength and power, but without the attendant muscle bulk. Competitive athletes who compete in weight limits are one example; wrestlers, MMA athletes, boxers, etc. Females are another group who, as a rule, want to get stronger when they train, but without adding much (or any) size. Some men desire steely, whip-like power but see the sheer weight of mass as non-functional—many martial artists fall into this category; perhaps Bruce Lee was the archetype.

But bodybuilders should also fall under this banner. All athletes who want to become as huge as possible need to spend some portion of their time focusing on *pure strength*. Without a high (and increasing) level of strength, it's impossible to use enough load to stress your muscles into getting bigger. This is even truer once you get past a certain basic point.

So: You want to build power like a Humvee, with the sleek lines of a classic Porsche? The following Ten Commandments have got you covered. Follow them, and we promise you *cannot* fail, even if you had trouble getting stronger in the past. Your days of weakness are done, my friend…

Enter the "Bullzelle"

There are guys who train for pure mass and want to look like bulls, and guys who only train for athleticism without mass, and are more like gazelles. Al Kavadlo has been described as a "bullzelle"—someone who trains mainly for strength, and has some muscle too, but without looking like a bulked-up bodybuilder. And guess what? It seems like many of the new generation of athletes want to be bullzelles! With Paul Wade's C-Mass program, you'll have what you need to achieve bullzelle looks and functionality should you want it...

COMMANDMENT I: Use low reps while keeping "fresh"!

If you want to generate huge strength without building muscle, here is the precise formula...

COMMANDMENT II: Utilize Hebb's Law—drill movements as often as possible!

How pure strength training works, in a nutshell...

Why frequency—how often you train—is often so radically different for *pure strength* trainers and for bodybuilders...

Training recipe for the perfect bodybuilder—and for the perfect strength trainer...

Why training for pure strength and training to *master a skill* are virtually identical methods.

COMMANDMENT III: Master muscle synergy!

If there is a "trick" to being supremely strong, THIS is it...

As a bodybuilder, are you making this huge mistake? If you want to get super-powerful, unlearn these ideas and employ THIS strategy instead...

Another great way to learn muscular coordination and control is to explore THESE drills...

COMMANDMENT IV: Brace Yourself!

If there is a single tactic that's *guaranteed* to maximize your body-power in short order, it's bracing. *Bracing* is both an art-form and a science. Here's how to do it and why it works so well.

COMMANDMENT V: Learn old-school breath control!

If there is an instant "trick" to increasing your strength, it's *learning the art of the breath*. Learn the details here...

Why inhalation is so important for strength and how to make it work most efficiently while lifting...

How the correctly-employed, controlled, forceful exhalation activates the muscles of the trunk, core and ribcage...

COMMANDMENT VI: Train your tendons!

When the old-time strongmen talked about strength, they rarely talked about muscle power—they typically focused on the integrity of the tendons. THIS is why...

The concept of "supple strength" and how to really train the *tendons* for optimal resilience and steely, real-life strength...

Why focusing on "peak contraction" can be devastating to your long-term strength-health goals...

COMMANDMENT VII: Focus on weak links!

THIS is the essential difference between a mere *bodybuilder* and a *truly powerful human being*...

Why focusing all your attention on the biggest, strongest muscle groups is counter-productive for developing your true strength potential...

Pay extra attention to your weakest areas by including THESE 4 sets of drills as a mandatory part of your monster strength program...

COMMANDMENT VIII: Exploit Neural Facilitation!

The nervous system—like most sophisticated biological systems—possesses different sets of *gears*. Learn how to safely and effectively shift to high gear in a hurry using THESE strategies...

COMMANDMENT IX: Apply Plyometric Patterns to Hack Neural Inhibition

Why it is fatal for a bodyweight master to focus only on tension-generating techniques and what to do instead...

How very fast movements can hugely increase your strength—the light bulb analogy.

The difference between "voluntary" and "involuntary" strength—and how to work on both for greater gains...

COMMANDMENT X: Master the power of the mind!

How to train the mind to make the body achieve incredible levels of strength and ferocity—as if it was tweaking on PCP...

5 fundamental ways to harness mental power and optimize your strength...

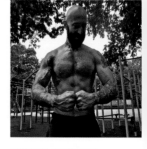

BONUS CHAPTER:
7. Supercharging Your Hormonal Profile

Why you should never, ever, ever take steroids to enhance your strength...

Hormones and muscle growth

Your *hormones* are what build your muscle. All your training is pretty secondary. You can work out hard as possible as often as possible, but if your hormonal levels aren't good, your gains will be close to nil. Learn what it takes to naturally optimize a cascade of powerful strength-generating hormones and to minimize the strength-sappers from sabotaging your gains...

Studies and simple experience have demonstrated that, far from being some esoteric practice, some men have increased their diminished total testosterone levels by *over a thousand percent*! How? Just by following a few basic rules.

What rules? Listen up. THIS is the most important bodybuilding advice anyone will ever give you.

The 6 Rules of Testosterone Building

THESE rules are the most powerful and long-lasting, for massive testosterone generation. Follow them if you want to get diesel.

The iron-clad case against steroid use and exogenous testosterone in general.

C-MASS
Calisthenics Mass: How To Maximize Muscle Growth Using Bodyweight-Only Training
By Paul "Coach" Wade

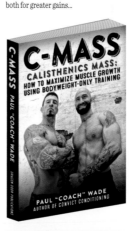

Book #B75 $24.95
eBook #EB75 $9.95
Paperback 8.5 x 11 • 136 pages, 130 pho[...]

How to Lead, Survive and Dominate Physically—And Reengineer Yourself As "The Complete Athletic Package"...

SUPERHUMAN POWER, MAXIMUM SPEED AND AGILITY, PLUS COMBAT-READY REFLEXES— USING BODYWEIGHT-ONLY METHODS

Explosive Calisthenics is for those who want to be winners and survivors in the game of life—for those who want to be the Complete Package: powerful, explosive, strong, agile, quick and resilient. Traditional martial arts have always understood this necessity of training the complete package—with explosive power at an absolute premium. And resilience is revered: the joints, tendons, muscles, organs and nervous system are ALL conditioned for maximum challenge.

Really great athletes are invariably that way too: agile as all get-go, blinding speed, ungodly bursts of power, superhuman displays of strength, seemingly at will...

The foundation and fundamentals center, first, around the building of power and speed. But *Explosive Calisthenics* does a masterful job of elucidating the skill-practices needed to safely prepare for and master the more ambitious moves.

But *Explosive Calisthenics* doesn't just inspire you with the dream of being the Complete Package. It gives you the complete blueprint, every detail and every progression you could possibly want and need to nail your dream and make it a reality. You, the Complete Package—it's all laid out for you, step by step

"The first physical attribute we lose as we age is our ability to generate power. Close behind is the loss of skilled, coordinated movement. The fix is never to lose these abilities in the first place! Paul Wade's "*Explosive Calisthenics* is the best program for developing power and skilled movement I have seen. Just as with his previous two books, the progressions are masterful with no fancy equipment needed. Do yourself a favor and get this amazing work. This book will be the gold standard for developing bodyweight power, skill, and agility."

—**CHRIS HARDY**, D.O. MPH, CSCS, author, *Strong Medicine*

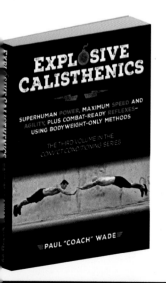

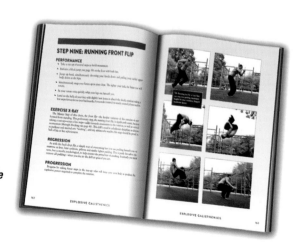

Explosive Calisthenics
Superhuman Power, Maximum Speed and Agility, Plus Combat-Ready Reflexes—Using Bodyweight-Only Methods
By Paul "Coach" Wade

Book #B80 $39.95
eBook #EB80 $19.95
Paperback 8.5 x 11
392 pages, 775 photos

> "**Explosive Calisthenics** is an absolute Treasure Map for anybody looking to tear down their body's athletic limitations. Who doesn't want to be able to kip to their feet from their back like a Bruce Lee? Or make a backflip look easy? Paul makes you want to put down the barbells, learn and practice these step-by-step progressions to mastering the most explosive and impressive bodyweight movements. The best part is? You can become an absolute Beast in under an hour of practice a week. Way to go, Paul! AROO!"
>
> —**Joe Distefano**, **Spartan Race**, Director of Training & Creator of the **Spartan SGX Certification**

— EXPLOSIVE CALISTHENICS —

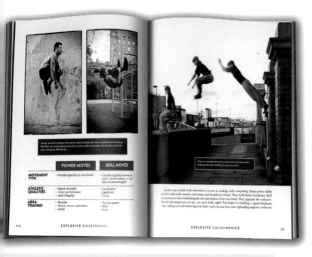

"Martial arts supremacy is all about explosive power and speed, and you will possess both once you've mastered the hardcore exercises in *Explosive Calisthenics*. Take your solo training to a level you never even imagined with these teeth-gritting, heart-palpating exercises—from a master of the genre."—**Loren W. Christensen**, author of over 50 books, including *Fighting Power: How to Develop Explosive Punches, Kicks, Blocks, And Grappling* and *Speed Training: How to Develop Your Maximum Speed for Martial Arts*

24 HOURS A DAY
ORDER NOW
1·800·899·5111
www.dragondoor.com

Order *Explosive Calisthenics* online:
www.dragondoor.com/b80

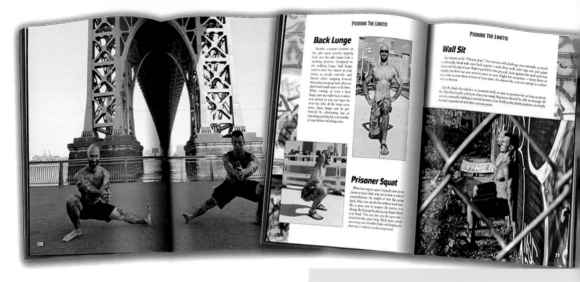

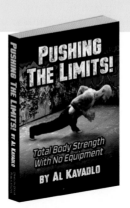

Sample Spreads From The Interior of *Stretching Your Boundaries*

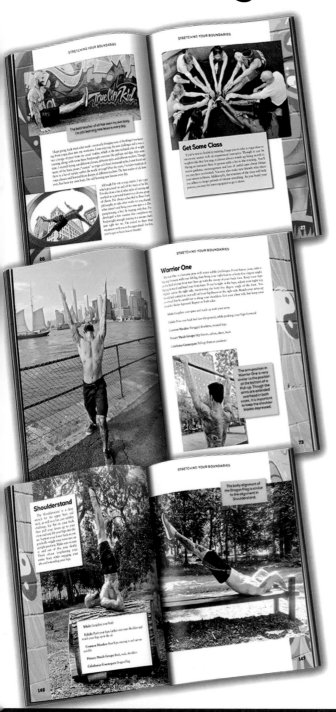

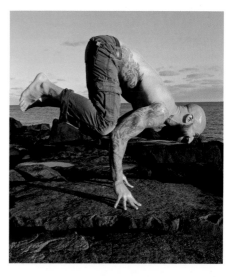

Stretching and Flexibility Secrets To Help Unlock Your Body—Be More Mobile, More Athletic, More Resilient And Far Stronger...

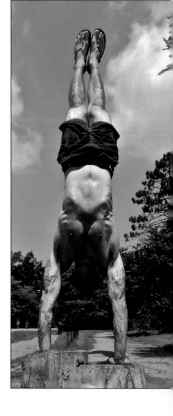

"The ultimate bodyweight mobility manual is here! Al Kavadlo's previous two Dragon Door books, **Raising the Bar** and **Pushing the Limits,** are the most valuable bodyweight strength training manuals in the world. But strength without mobility is meaningless. Al has used his many years of training and coaching to fuse bodyweight disciplines such as yoga, martial arts, rehabilitative therapy and bar athletics into the ultimate calisthenics stretching compendium. **Stretching your Boundaries** belongs on the shelf of any serious athlete—it's bodyweight mobility dynamite!"

—**"COACH" PAUL WADE, author of** *Convict Conditioning*

"In this book, Al invites you to take a deeper look at the often overlooked, and sometimes demonized, ancient practice of static stretching. He wrestles with many of the questions, dogmas and flat out lies about stretching that have plagued the fitness practitioner for at least the last decade. And finally he gives you a practical guide to static stretching that will improve your movement, performance, breathing and life. In **Stretching Your Boundaries,** you'll sense Al's deep understanding and love for the human body. Thank you Al, for helping to bring awareness to perhaps the most important aspect of physical education and fitness."

—**ELLIOTT HULSE, creator of the** *Grow Stronger* **method**

"An absolutely masterful follow up to **Raising The Bar** and **Pushing The Limits,** Stretching Your Boundaries really completes the picture. Both easy to understand and fully applicable, Al's integration of traditional flexibility techniques with his own unique spin makes this a must have. The explanation of how each stretch will benefit your calisthenics practice is brilliant. Not only stunning in its color and design, this book also gives you the true feeling of New York City, both gritty and euphoric, much like Al's personality."

—**MIKE FITCH, creator of Global Bodyweight Training**

"Stretching Your Boundaries is a terrific resource that will unlock your joints so you can build more muscle, strength and athleticism. Al's passion for human performance radiates in this beautifully constructed book. Whether you're stiff as a board, or an elite gymnast, this book outlines the progressions to take your body and performance to a new level."

—**CHAD WATERBURY, M.S., author of** *Huge in a Hurry*

"Al Kavadlo has done it again! He's created yet another incredible resource that I wish I had twenty years ago. Finding great material on flexibility training that actually enhances your strength is like trying to find a needle in a haystack. But look no further, because **Stretching Your Boundaries** is exactly what you need."

—**JASON FERRUGGIA, Strength Coach**

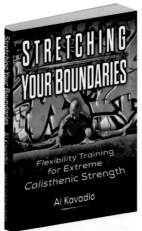

Stretching Your Boundaries
Flexibility Training for Extreme Calisthenic Strength
By Al Kavadlo

Book #B73 $39.95
eBook # EB73 $19.9
Paperback 8.5 x 11
214 pages • 235 photos

How Do YOU Stack Up Against These 6 Signs of a TRUE Physical Specimen?

According to Paul Wade's Convict Conditioning you earn the right to call yourself a 'true physical specimen' if you can perform the following:

1. **AT LEAST** one set of 5 one-arm pushups each side—with the ELITE goal of 100 sets each side

2. **AT LEAST** one set of 5 one-leg squats each side—with the ELITE goal of 2 sets of 50 each side

3. **AT LEAST** a single one-arm pullup each side—with the ELITE goal of 2 sets of 6 each side

4. **AT LEAST** one set of 5 hanging straight leg raises—with the ELITE goal of 2 sets of 30

5. **AT LEAST** one stand-to-stand bridge—with the ELITE goal of 2 sets of 30

Well, how DO you stack up?

Chances are that whatever athletic level you have achieved, there are some serious gaps in your OVERALL strength program. Gaps that stop you short of being able to claim status as a truly accomplished strength athlete.

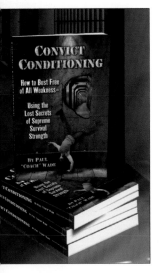

The good news is that—in *Convict Conditioning*—Paul Wade has laid out a brilliant 6-set system of 10 progressions which allows you to master these elite levels.

And you could be starting at almost any age and in almost in any condition...

Paul Wade has given you the keys—ALL the keys you'll ever need— that will open door, after door, after door for you in your quest for supreme physical excellence. Yes, it will be the hardest work you'll ever have to do. And yes, 97% of those who pick up *Convict Conditioning*, frankly, won't have the guts and the fortitude to make it. But if you make it even half-way through **Paul's Progressions**, you'll be stronger than almost anyone you encounter. Ever.

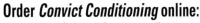

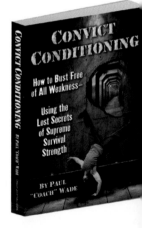

Dragon Door Customer Acclaim for Paul Wade's Convict Conditioning

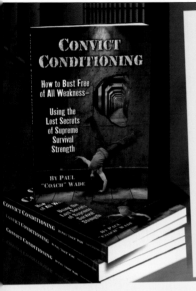

A Strength Training Guide That Will Never Be Duplicated!

"I knew within the first chapter of reading this book that I was in for something special and unique. The last time I felt this same feeling was when reading *Power to the People!* To me this is the Body Weight equivalent to Pavel's masterpiece.

Books like this can never be duplicated. Paul Wade went through a unique set of circumstances of doing time in prison with an 'old time' master of calisthenics. Paul took these lessons from this 70 year old strong man and mastered them over a period of 20 years while 'doing time'. He then taught these methods to countless prisoners and honed his teaching to perfection.

I believe that extreme circumstances like this are what it takes to create a true masterpiece. I know that 'masterpiece' is a strong word, but this is as close as it gets. No other body weight book I have read (and I have a huge fitness library)...comes close to this as far as gaining incredible strength from body weight exercise.

Just like Power to the People, I am sure I will read this over and over again...mastering the principles that Paul Wade took 20 years to master.

Outstanding Book!"—*Rusty Moore - Fitness Black Book - Seattle, WA*

A must for all martial artists

As a dedicated martial artist for more than seven years, this book is exactly what I've been looking for.

For a while now I have trained with machines at my local gym to improve my muscle strength and power and get to the next level in my training. I always felt that the modern health club, technology based exercise jarred with my martial art though, which only required body movement.

Finally this book has come along. At last I can combine perfect body movement for martial skill with perfect body exercise for ultimate strength.

All fighting arts are based on body movement. This book is a complete textbook on how to max out your musclepower using only body movement, as different from dumbbells, machines or gadgets. For this reason it belongs on the bookshelf of every serious martial artist, male and female, young and old."—*Gino Cartier - Washington DC*

I've packed all of my other training books away!

I read CC in one go. I couldn't put it down. I have purchased a lot of bodyweight training books in the past, and have always been pretty disappointed. They all seem to just have pictures of different exercises, and no plan whatsoever on how to implement them and progress with them. But not with this one. The information in this book is AWESOME! I like to have a clear, logical plan of progression to follow, and that is what this book gives. I have put all of my other training books away. CC is the only system I am going to follow. This is now my favorite training book ever!"—*Lyndan - Australia*

Brutal Elegance.

"I have been training and reading about training since I first joined the US Navy in the 1960s. I thought I'd seen everything the fitness world had to offer. Sometimes twice. But I was wrong. This book is utterly iconoclastic.

The author breaks down all conceivable body weight exercises into six basic movements, each designed to stimulate different vectors of the muscular system. These six are then elegantly and very intelligently broken into ten progressive techniques. You master one technique, and move on to the next.

The simplicity of this method belies a very powerful and complex training paradigm, reduced into an abstraction that obviously took many years of sweat and toil to develop. Trust me. Nobody else worked this out. This approach is completely unique and fresh.

I have read virtually every calisthenics book printed in America over the last 40 years, and instruction like this can't be found anywhere, in any one of them. *Convict Conditioning* is head and shoulders above them all. In years to come, trainers and coaches will all be talking about 'progressions' and 'progressive calisthenics' and claim they've been doing it all along. But the truth is that Dragon Door bought it to you first. As with kettlebells, they were the trail blazers.

Who should purchase this volume? Everyone who craves fitness and strength should. Even if you don't plan to follow the routines, the book will make you think about your physical prowess, and will give even world class experts food for thought. At the very least if you find yourself on vacation or away on business without your barbells, this book will turn your hotel into a fully equipped gym.

I'd advise any athlete to obtain this work as soon as possible."
—*Bill Oliver - Albany, NY, United States*

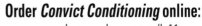

More Dragon Door Customer Acclaim for Convict Conditioning

Fascinating Reading and Real Strength

"Coach Wade's system is a real eye opener if you've been a lifetime iron junkie. Wanna find out how really strong (or weak) you are? Get this book and begin working through the 10 levels of the 6 power exercises. I was pleasantly surprised by my ability on a few of the exercises...but some are downright humbling. If I were on a desert island with only one book on strength and conditioning this would be it. (Could I staple Pavel's "Naked Warrior" to the back and count them as one???!) Thanks Dragon Door for this innovative new author."—*Jon Schultheis, RKC (2005) - Keansburg, NJ*

Single best strength training book ever!

"I just turned 50 this year and I have tried a little bit of everything over the years: martial arts, swimming, soccer, cycling, free weights, weight machines, even yoga and Pilates. I started using *Convict Conditioning* right after it came out. I started from the beginning, like Coach Wade says, doing mostly step one or two for five out of the six exercises. I work out 3 to 5 times a week, usually for 30 to 45 minutes.

Long story short, my weight went up 14 pounds (I was not trying to gain weight) but my body fat percentage dropped two percent. That translates into approximately 19 pounds of lean muscle gained in two months! I've never gotten this kind of results with anything else I've ever done. Now I have pretty much stopped lifting weights for strength training. Instead, I lift once a week as a test to see how much stronger I'm getting without weight training. There are a lot of great strength training books in the world (most of them published by Dragon Door), but if I had to choose just one, this is the single best strength training book ever. BUY THIS BOOK. FOLLOW THE PLAN. GET AS STRONG AS YOU WANT. "—*Wayne - Decatur, GA*

Best bodyweight training book so far!

"I'm a martial artist and I've been training for years with a combination of weights and bodyweight training and had good results from both (but had the usual injuries from weight training). I prefer the bodyweight stuff though as it trains me to use my whole body as a unit, much more than weights do, and I notice the difference on the mat and in the ring. Since reading this book I have given the weights a break and focused purely on the bodyweight exercise progressions as described by 'Coach' Wade and my strength had increased more than ever before. So far I've built up to 12 strict one-leg squats each leg and 5 uneven pull ups each arm.

I've never achieved this kind of strength before - and this stuff builds solid muscle mass as well. It's very intense training. I am so confident in and happy with the results I'm getting that I've decided to train for a fitness/bodybuilding comp just using his techniques, no weights, just to show for real what kind of a physique these exercises can build. In sum, I cannot recommend 'Coach' Wade's book highly enough - it is by far the best of its kind ever!"—*Mark Robinson - Australia, currently living in South Korea*

A lifetime of lifting...and continued learning.

"I have been working out diligently since 1988 and played sports in high school and college before that. My stint in the Army saw me doing calisthenics, running, conditioning courses, forced marches, etc. There are many levels of strength and fitness. I have been as big as 240 in my powerlifting/strongman days and as low as 185-190 while in the Army. I think I have tried everything under the sun: the high intensity of Arthur Jones and Dr. Ken, the Super Slow of El Darden, and the brutality of Dinosaur Training Brooks Kubic made famous.

This is one of the BEST books I've ever read on real strength training which also covers other just as important aspects of health; like staying injury free, feeling healthy and becoming flexible. It's an excellent book. He tells you the why and the how with his progressive plan. This book is a GOLD MINE and worth 100 times what I paid for it!"
—*Horst - Woburn, MA*

This book sets the standard, ladies and gentlemen

"It's difficult to describe just how much this book means to me. I've been training hard since I was in the RAF nearly ten years ago, and to say this book is a breakthrough is an understatement. How often do you really read something so new, so fresh? This book contains a complete new system of calisthenics drawn from American prison training methods. When I say 'system' I mean it. It's complete (rank beginner to expert), it's comprehensive (all the exercises and photos are here), it's graded (progressions from exercise to exercise are smooth and pre-determined) and it's totally original. Whether you love or hate the author, you have to listen to him. And you will learn something. This book just makes SENSE. In twenty years people will still be buying it."—Andy McMann - Ponty, Wales, GB

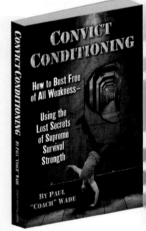

Convict Conditioning

How to Bust Free of All Weakness— Using the Lost Secrets of Supreme Survival Strength
By Paul "Coach" Wade

Book #B41 $39.95
eBook #EB41 $19.95
Paperback 8.5 x 11
320 pages • 191 photos

The Experts Give High Praise to
Convict Conditioning 2

"Coach Paul Wade has outdone himself. His first book *Convict Conditioning* is to my mind THE BEST book ever written on bodyweight conditioning. Hands down. Now, with the sequel *Convict Conditioning 2*, Coach Wade takes us even deeper into the subtle nuances of training with the ultimate resistance tool: our bodies.

In plain English, but with an amazing understanding of anatomy, physiology, kinesiology and, go figure, psychology, Coach Wade explains very simply how to work the smaller but just as important areas of the body such as the hands and forearms, neck and calves and obliques in serious functional ways.

His minimalist approach to exercise belies the complexity of his system and the deep insight into exactly how the body works and the best way to get from A to Z in the shortest time possible.

I got the best advice on how to strengthen the hard-to-reach extensors of the hand right away from this exercise Master I have ever seen. It's so simple but so completely functional I can't believe no one else has thought of it yet. Just glad he figured it out for me.

Paul teaches us how to strengthen our bodies with the simplest of movements while at the same time balancing our structures in the same way: simple exercises that work the whole body.

And just as simply as he did with his first book. His novel approach to stretching and mobility training is brilliant and fresh as well as his take on recovery and healing from injury. Sprinkled throughout the entire book are too-many-to-count insights and advice from a man who has come to his knowledge the hard way and knows exactly of what he speaks.

This book is, as was his first, an amazing journey into the history of physical culture disguised as a book on calisthenics. But the thing that Coach Wade does better than any before him is his unbelievable progressions on EVERY EXERCISE and stretch! He breaks things down and tells us EXACTLY how to proceed to get to whatever level of strength and development we want. AND gives us the exact metrics we need to know when to go to the next level.

Adding in completely practical and immediately useful insights into nutrition and the mindset necessary to deal not only with training but with life, makes this book a classic that will stand the test of time.

Bravo Coach Wade, Bravo." —**Mark Reifkind, Master RKC,** author of *Mastering the HardStyle Kettlebell Swing*

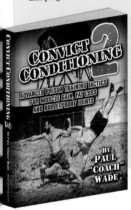

Convict Conditioning 2
Advanced Prison Training Tactics for Muscle Gain, Fat Loss and Bulletproof Joints
By Paul "Coach" Wade

Book #B59 $39.95
eBook #EB59 $19.95
Paperback 8.5 x 11
354 pages • 261 photos

"The overriding principle of *Convict Conditioning* 2 is 'little equipment-big rewards'. For the athlete in the throwing and fighting arts, the section on Lateral Chain Training, Capturing the Flag, is a unique and perhaps singular approach to training the obliques and the whole family of side muscles. This section stood out to me as ground breaking and well worth the time and energy by anyone to review and attempt to complete. Literally, this is a new approach to lateral chain training that is well beyond sidebends and suitcase deadlifts.

The author's review of passive stretching reflects the experience of many of us in the field. But, his solution might be the reason I am going to recommend this work for everyone: The Trifecta. This section covers what the author calls The Functional Triad and gives a series of simple progressions to three holds that promise to oil your joints. It's yoga for the strength athlete and supports the material one would find, for example, in Pavel's *Loaded Stretching*.

I didn't expect to like this book, but I come away from it practically insisting that everyone read it. It is a strongman book mixed with yoga mixed with street smarts. I wanted to hate it, but I love it."
—**Dan John,** author of *Don't Let Go* and co-author of *Easy Strength*

"I've been lifting weights for over 50 years and have trained in the martial arts since 1965. I've read voraciously on both subjects, and written dozens of magazine articles and many books on the subjects. This book and Wade's first, *Convict Conditioning*, are by far the most commonsense, information-packed, and result producing I've read. These books will truly change your life.

Paul Wade is a new and powerful voice in the strength and fitness arena, one that is commonsense, inspiring, and in your face. His approach to maximizing your body's potential is not the same old hackneyed material you find in every book and magazine piece that pictures steroid-bloated models screaming as they curl weights. Wade's stuff has been proven effective by hard men who don't tolerate fluff. It will work for you, too—guaranteed.

As an ex-cop, I've gone mano-y-mano with ex-cons that had clearly trained as Paul Wade suggests in his two *Convict Conditioning* books. While these guys didn't look like steroid-fueled bodybuilders (actually, there were a couple who did), all were incredibly lean, hard and powerful. Wade blows many commonly held beliefs about conditioning, strengthening, and eating out of the water and replaces them with result-producing information that won't cost you a dime." —**Loren W. Christensen,** author of *Fighting the Pain Resistant Attacker,* and many other titles

"*Convict Conditioning* is one of the most influential books I ever got my hands on. *Convict Conditioning 2* took my training and outlook on the power of bodyweight training to the 10th degree—from strengthening the smallest muscles in a maximal manner, all the way to using bodyweight training as a means of healing injuries that pile up from over 22 years of aggressive lifting.

I've used both *Convict Conditioning* and *Convict Conditioning 2* on myself and with my athletes. Without either of these books I can easily say that these boys would not be the BEASTS they are today. Without a doubt *Convict Conditioning 2* will blow you away and inspire and educate you to take bodyweight training to a whole NEW level."
—**Zach Even-Esh,** Underground Strength Coach

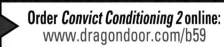

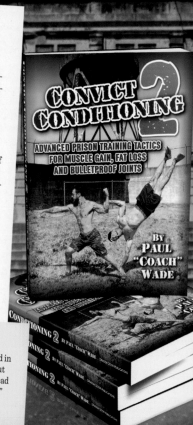

—TABLE OF CONTENTS—

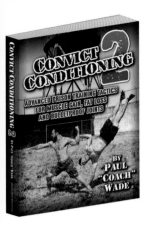

Convict Conditioning 2
Advanced Prison Training Tactics for Muscle Gain, Fat Loss and Bulletproof Joints
By Paul "Coach" Wade

Book #B59 $39.95
eBook #EB59 $19.95
Paperback 8.5 x 11
354 pages • 261 photos

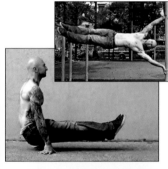

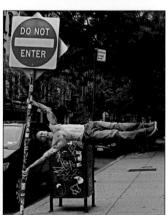

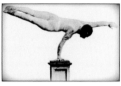
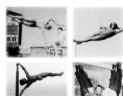
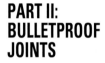
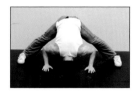
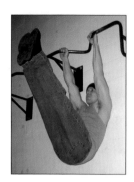
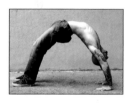
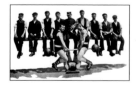
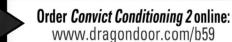

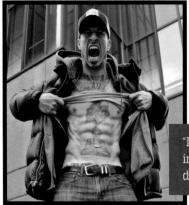

Are You Dissatisfied With Your Abs?

"Diamond-Cut Abs condenses decades of agonizing lessons and insight into the best book on ab-training ever written. Hands down." —**PAUL WADE**, author of *Convict Conditioning*

Are you dissatisfied with your abs? Does it seem a distant dream for you to own a rock-solid center? Can you only hanker in vain for the chiseled magnificence of a Greek statue? Have you given up on owning the tensile functionality and explosive power of a cage-fighter's core?

According to Danny Kavadlo, training your abs is a whole-life endeavor. It's about right eating, right drinking, right rest, right practice, right exercise at the right time, right motivation, right inspiration, right attitude and right lifestyle. If you don't have that righteous set of abs in place, it's because you have failed in one or more of these areas.

With his 25-plus years of rugged research and extreme physical dedication into every dimension of what it takes to earn world-class abs, Danny Kavadlo is a modern-day master of the art. It's all here: over 50 of the best-ever exercises to develop the abs—from beginner to superman level—inspirational photos, no BS straight talk on nutrition and lifestyle factors and clear-cut instructions on what to do, when. Supply the grit, follow the program and you simply cannot fail but to build a monstrous mid-section.

In our culture, Abs are the Measure of a Man. To quit on your abs is to quit on your masculinity—like it or not. *Diamond-Cut Abs* gives you the complete, whole-life program you need to reassert yourself and reestablish your respect as a true physical specimen—with a thunderous six-pack to prove it.

Are You Dissatisfied With Your Abs?

In the Abs Gospel According to Danny, training your abs is a whole-life endeavor. It's about right eating, right drinking, right rest, right practice, right exercise at the right time, right motivation, right inspiration, right attitude and right lifestyle.

So, yes, all of this Rightness gets covered in *Diamond-Cut Abs*. But let's not confuse Right with Rigid. Apprentice in the Danny School of Abs and it's like apprenticing with a world-class Chef—a mix of incredible discipline, inspired creativity and a passionate love-affair with your art.

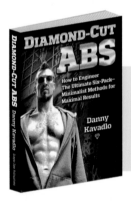

"Danny has done it again! *Diamond-Cut Abs* is a no-nonsense, results driven approach that delivers all the goods on abs. Nutrition, training and progression are all included, tattoos optional!"— ROBB WOLF, author of *The Paleo Solution*

"There are a lot of abs books and products promising a six-pack. What sets Danny's book apart is the realistic and reasonable first section of the book... His insights into nutrition are so simple and sound, there is a moment you wish this book was a stand alone dieting book."—DAN JOHN, author of *Never Let Go*

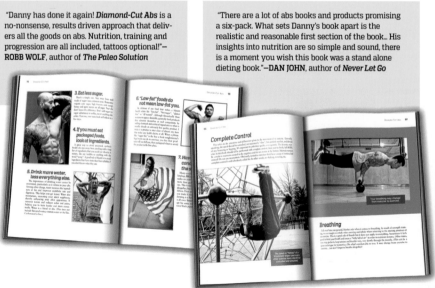

Diamond-Cut Abs
How to Engineer the Ultimate Six-Pack— Minimalist Methods for Maximum Results
By Danny Kavadlo

Book #B77 $39.95
eBook #EB77 $19.95
Paperback 8.5 x 11
230 pages, 305 photos

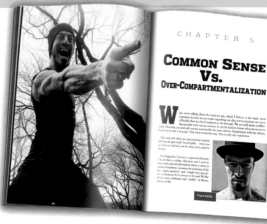

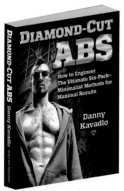

Diamond-Cut Abs
How to Engineer the Ultimate Six-Pack— Minimalist Methods for Maximum Results
By Danny Kavadlo

Book #B77 $39.95
eBook #EB77 $19.95
Paperback 8.5 x 11
230 pages, 305 photos

Reader Praise for *Convict Conditioning Ultimate Bodyweight Training Log*

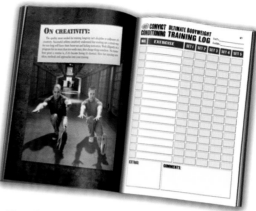

Above and Beyond!

"Not JUST a log book. TONS of great and actually useful info. I really like to over complicate programming and data entries at times. And honestly, All one has to do is fill in the blanks... Well that and DO THE WORK. Great product."
—NOEL PRICE, Chicagoland, IL

A unique training log

"This log book is one of a kind in the world. It is the only published body weight exclusive training log I have personally seen. It is well structured and provides everything for a log book in a primarily body weight oriented routine. The book is best integrated with the other books in the convict conditioning series however has enough information to act as a stand alone unit. It is a must have for anyone who is a fan of the convict conditioning series or is entering into calisthenics."
—CARTER D., Cambridge, Canada

Excellent Companion to *Convict Conditioning 1 & 2*

"This is an amazing book! If you are a fan of Convict Conditioning (1 & 2) you need to get this training log. If you are preparing for the Progressive Calisthenics Certification then it's a must-have!!! The spiral bound format is a huge improvement over the regular binding and it makes it that much more functional for use in the gym. Great design, amazing pictures and additional content! Once again - Great job Dragon Door!"
—MICHAEL KRIVKA, RKC Team Leader, Gaithersburg, MD

Excellent latest addition to the CC Program!

"A terrific book to keep you on track and beyond. Thank you again for this incredible series!"
—JOSHUA HATCHER, Holyoke, MA

Calling this a Log Book is Selling it Short

"I thought, what is the big deal about a logbook! Seriously mistaken. It is a work of art and with tips on each page that would be a great book all by itself. Get it. It goes way beyond a log book...the logging part of this book is just a bonus. You must have this!"**—JON ENGUM, Brainerd, MN**

The Ultimate Bodyweight Conditioning

"I have started to incorporate bodyweight training into my strength building when I am not going to the gym. At the age of 68, after 30 years in the gym the 'Convict Conditioning Log' is going to be a welcome new training challenge."
—WILLIAM HAYDEN, Winter Park, FL

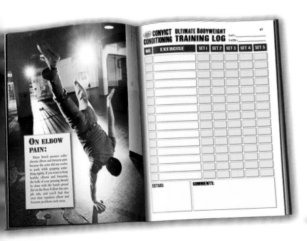

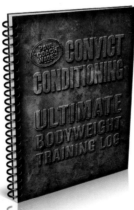

Convict Conditioning Ultimate Bodyweight Training Log
By Paul "Coach" Wade

Book #B67 $29.95
eBook #EB67 $19.95
Paperback (spiral bound) 6 x 9
290 pages • 175 photos

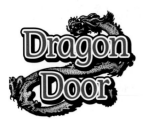

1•800•899•5111 • 24HOURS

FAX YOUR ORDER (866) 280-7619

O R D E R I N G   I N F O R M A T I O N

Telephone Orders For faster service you may place your orders by calling Toll Free 24 hours a day, 7 days a week, 365 days per year. When you call, please have your credit card ready.

Customer Service Questions? Please call us between 9:00am– 11:00pm EST Monday to Friday at 1-800-899-5111. Local and foreign customers call 513-346-4160 for orders and customer service

100% One-Year Risk-Free Guarantee. If you are not completely satisfied with any product—we'll be happy to give you a prompt exchange, credit, or refund, as you wish. Simply return your purchase to us, and please let us know why you were dissatisfied--it will help us to provide better products and services in the future. Shipping and handling fees are non-refundable.

COMPLETE AND MAIL WITH FULL PAYMENT TO: DRAGON DOOR PUBLICATIONS, 5 COUNTY ROAD B EAST, SUITE 3, LITTLE CANADA, MN 55117

Please print clearly

Sold To:

A

Name_____

Street_____

City_____

State _____ Zip _____

Please print clearly

Sold To: (Street address for delivery)   **B**

Name_____

Street _____

City _____

State _____ Zip _____

Email_____

WARNING TO FOREIGN CUSTOMERS:

The Customs in your country may or may not tax or otherwise charge you an additional fee for goods you receive. Dragon Door Publications is charging you only for U.S. handling and international shipping. Dragon Door Publications is in no way responsible for any additional fees levied by Customs, the carrier or any other entity.

Item #	Qty.	Item Description	Item Price	A or B	Total

HANDLING AND SHIPPING CHARGES • NO CODS

Total Amount of Order Add (Excludes kettlebells and kettlebell kits):

$00.00 to 29.99	Add $7.00	$100.00 to 129.99	Add $14.00
$30.00 to 49.99	Add $6.00	$130.00 to 169.99	Add $16.00
$50.00 to 69.99	Add $8.00	$170.00 to 199.99	Add $18.00
$70.00 to 99.99	Add $11.00	$200.00 to 299.99	Add $20.00
		$300.00 and up	Add $24.00

Canada and Mexico add $6.00 to US charges. All other countries, flat rate, double US Charges. See Kettlebell section for Kettlebell Shipping and handling charges.

Total of Goods	
Shipping Charges	
Rush Charges	
Kettlebell Shipping Charges	
OH residents add 6.5%	
sales tax	
MN residents add 6.5% sales	

METHOD OF PAYMENT ____Check ____M.O. ____Mastercard ____Visa ____Discover ____Amex

Account No. (Please indicate all the numbers on your credit card)   EXPIRATION DATE

☐☐☐☐ ☐☐☐☐ ☐☐☐☐ ☐☐☐☐   ☐☐/☐☐

Day Phone: _____

Signature: _____   Date: _____

NOTE: We ship best method available for your delivery address. Foreign orders are sent by air. Credit card or International M.O. only. **For RUSH processing** of your order, add an additional $10.00 per address. Available on money order & charge card orders only.

Errors and omissions excepted. Prices subject to change without notice.

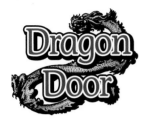

1•800•899•5111 • 24HOURS
FAX YOUR ORDER (866) 280-7619
O R D E R I N G   I N F O R M A T I O N

Telephone Orders For faster service you may place your orders by calling Toll Free 24 hours a day, 7 days a week, 365 days per year. When you call, please have your credit card ready.

Customer Service Questions? Please call us between 9:00am– 11:00pm EST Monday to Friday at 1-800-899-5111. Local and foreign customers call 513-346-4160 for orders and customer service

100% One-Year Risk-Free Guarantee. If you are not completely satisfied with any product—we'll be happy to give you a prompt exchange, credit, or refund, as you wish. Simply return your purchase to us, and please let us know why you were dissatisfied--it will help us to provide better products and services in the future. Shipping and handling fees are non-refundable.

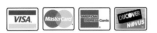

COMPLETE AND MAIL WITH FULL PAYMENT TO: DRAGON DOOR PUBLICATIONS, 5 COUNTY ROAD B EAST, SUITE 3, LITTLE CANADA, MN 55117

Please print clearly
Sold To:

A

Name_____

Street_____

City_____

State _____ Zip _____

Please print clearly
Sold To: (Street address for delivery)   **B**

Name_____

Street _____

City _____

State _____ Zip _____

Email_____

WARNING TO FOREIGN CUSTOMERS:

The Customs in your country may or may not tax or otherwise charge you an additional fee for goods you receive. Dragon Door Publications is charging you only for U.S. handling and international shipping. Dragon Door Publications is in no way responsible for any additional fees levied by Customs, the carrier or any other entity.

ITEM #	QTY.	ITEM DESCRIPTION	ITEM PRICE	A OR B	TOTAL

HANDLING AND SHIPPING CHARGES • NO CODS
Total Amount of Order Add (Excludes kettlebells and kettlebell kits):

$00.00 to 29.99	Add $7.00	$100.00 to 129.99	Add $14.00
$30.00 to 49.99	Add $6.00	$130.00 to 169.99	Add $16.00
$50.00 to 69.99	Add $8.00	$170.00 to 199.99	Add $18.00
$70.00 to 99.99	Add $11.00	$200.00 to 299.99	Add $20.00
		$300.00 and up	Add $24.00

Canada and Mexico add $6.00 to US charges. All other countries, flat rate, double US Charges. See Kettlebell section for Kettlebell Shipping and handling charges.

Total of Goods	
Shipping Charges	
Rush Charges	
Kettlebell Shipping Charges	
OH residents add 6.5%	
sales tax	
MN residents add 6.5% sales	

METHOD OF PAYMENT ___CHECK ___M.O. ___MASTERCARD ___VISA ___DISCOVER ___AMEX

Account No. (Please indicate all the numbers on your credit card)   EXPIRATION DATE

▢▢▢▢ ▢▢▢▢ ▢▢▢▢ ▢▢▢▢   ▢▢/▢▢

Day Phone: _____

Signature: _____ Date: _____

NOTE: We ship best method available for your delivery address. Foreign orders are sent by air. Credit card or International M.O. only. **For RUSH processing** of your order, add an additional $10.00 per address. Available on money order & charge card orders only.

Errors and omissions excepted. Prices subject to change without notice.